HEALTH CARE, ETHICS AND INSURANCE

Health Care, Ethics and Insurance presents a timely and provocative examination of the ethical implications of health insurance, which draws on the most recent scientific developments, legislation and trends in political economy.

The volume is divided into two main parts. The first considers the ethics of underwriting, that is, the ethics of risk assessment and the acceptance and refusal of insurance risk by insurers, and considers the treatment by insurers of high-risk applicants, including those who are HIV+, who have genetic disorders or who are disabled. Part II examines the arguments for a mix of public and private insurance for acute and long-term care, as well as income protection insurance after retirement from work.

This comprehensive and controversial book provides an essential survey of the key issues in health insurance as well as recommendations for improvement.

Tom Sorell is Professor of Philosophy, University of Essex. He is principal author of *Business Ethics* (1994) and is Associate Editor of *Business Ethics: A European Review*.

PROFESSIONAL ETHICS
General editor: Ruth Chadwick
*Centre for Professional Ethics,
University of Central Lancashire*

Professionalism is a subject of interest to academics, the general public and would-be professional groups. Traditional ideas of professions and professional conduct have been challenged by recent social, political and technological changes. One result has been the development for almost every profession of an ethical code of conduct which attempts to formalise its values and standards. These codes of conduct raise questions about the status of a 'profession' and the consequent moral implications for behaviour.

This series seeks to examine these questions both critically and constructively. Individual volumes consider issues relevant to particular professions, including nursing, genetic counselling, journalism, business, the food industry and law. Other volumes address issues relevant to all professional groups, such as the function and value of a code of ethics and the demands of confidentiality.

Also available in this series:
ETHICAL ISSUES IN JOURNALISM AND THE MEDIA
edited by Andrew Belsey and Ruth Chadwick

GENETIC COUNSELLING
edited by Angus Clarke

ETHICAL ISSUES IN NURSING
edited by Geoffrey Hunt

THE GROUND OF PROFESSIONAL ETHICS
Daryl Koehn

ETHICAL ISSUES IN SOCIAL WORK
edited by Richard Hugman and David Smith

FOOD ETHICS
edited by Ben Mepham

CURRENT ISSUES IN BUSINESS ETHICS
edited by Peter W. F. Davies

THE ETHICS OF BANKRUPTCY
Jukka Kilpi

HEALTH CARE, ETHICS AND INSURANCE

Edited by Tom Sorell

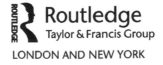

LONDON AND NEW YORK

First published 1998
by Routledge
2 Park Square, Milton Park, Abingdon, Oxon, OX14 4RN
Simultaneously published in the USA and Canada
by Routledge
711 Third Avenue, New York, NY 10017

Typeset in Times by
BC Typesetting, Bristol

Routledge is an imprint of the Taylor & Francis Group, an informa business

British Library Cataloguing in Publication Data
A catalogue record for this book is available from the British Library

Library of Congress Cataloging in Publication Data
Health care, ethics and insurance/edited by Tom Sorell.
p.   cm. – (Professional ethics)
1. Medical care – Great Britain.   2. Medical ethics – Great Britain.
3. Insurance, Health – Great Britain.   I. Sorell, Tom.   II. Series.
RA395.G6H38   1998
362.1′0941–dc21   98-13842
                                  CIP

ISBN 13: 978-0-415-16284-5 (hbk)
ISBN 13: 978-0-415-16285-2 (pbk)

To the memory of David Cavers

CONTENTS

CONTENTS

CONTENTS

CONTENTS

TABLES

CONTRIBUTORS

Philip M. Booth is Senior Lecturer in Actuarial Science, City University, London.

Will Cartwright is a Lecturer in Philosophy, University of Essex.

David Cavers died in 1997. He was Managing Director of Norwich Union Healthcare.

Stephen Diacon is Senior Lecturer in Insurance and Director of the Insurance Centre at the University of Nottingham.

Gerry M. Dickinson is Professor of International Insurance and Director of the Centre for Insurance and Investment Studies, City University Business School, London.

Heather Draper is Lecturer in Biomedical Ethics, University of Birmingham.

Paul Fenn is Norwich Union Professor of Insurance Studies, University of Nottingham.

Philippa Gannon is Lecturer in Law, University of Glasgow.

Spencer Leigh is a director of Worldwide Reassurance and a consultant underwriter for Royal Liver Insurance.

Sheila A. M. McLean is International Bar Association Professor of Law and Ethics in Medicine, University of Glasgow.

Peter G. Moore is Emeritus Professor of Decision Sciences, London Business School.

Tom Sorell is Professor of Philosophy, University of Essex.

Albert Weale is Professor of Government, University of Essex.

ACKNOWLEDGEMENTS

For Chapter 3, 'Genetics and ethics', the Medical Research Council of Great Britain, item HCP 41, Science and Technology Select Committee, Third Report, *Human Genetics*, parliamentary copyright; reproduced with the permission of the Controller of Her Majesty's Stationery Office. Chapter 10, 'Public or private?', Parts Two and Three of *The Insurance Solution*, European Policy Forum pamphlet (London, 1997); reprinted by permission of the European Policy Forum.

INTRODUCTION

The questions considered in this book are made timely by both recent science and recent political economy. Health insurance in general and cover for certain serious diseases in particular are directly affected by advances in medical research. For example, drug therapies for AIDS now allow sufferers to keep their jobs and lead lives outside hospital: the risks to insurers of life and health insurance claims from AIDS have had to be reconsidered as a result. Markers of certain inherited diseases can now be identified by tests devised by geneticists. Should insurers have access to the results of these tests, if people with the unwanted markers end up being ineligible for affordable health care? These are among the ethical questions raised by recent science. The relevant developments in political economy are associated with the soaring costs of funding the welfare state, and the general reluctance of political parties and their electorates to raise the extra money from direct taxation. The cost not only of public health services but also of social services and pensions has to be considered in this connection. To meet the cost, large Western European welfare states may have to encourage individuals to insure themselves for long-term care and contribute directly to their own pension schemes. Perhaps contracts between public health authorities and private medical insurers will also have to be considered as a source of funding for capital projects and services within public sector health services. The major ethical question here is whether privatising pensions or care for the elderly or more of mainstream medical insurance will leave anyone with no safety net, or too many people with an inadequate safety net. As is well known from the case of the US, the money costs and moral costs of a system of non-compulsory, mainly private insurance can be very large, and these costs are just as real for those who are wondering how to reduce a vast welfare state to a manageable size as for those who have a welfare state that is too minimal to meet the demands placed upon it.

Urgent as it is to answer ethical questions about insurance, the literature devoted to them in their timely forms is not extensive, and is often geared to social and economic assumptions appropriate to the United States.[1] The questions raised in this book are clearly central to health care as a public policy issue and to health care as an important and growing sector of business activity in the developed world, and so they ought to register as important in more than one sector of applied or professional ethics. The fact that they are relatively undiscussed may be more a reflection of the number of different sectors of health care and business and policy that they engage than of lack of interest in them. To do justice in this volume to the many dimensions of the issues considered, it has been necessary to enlist contributors from an unusually wide range of backgrounds. Two of the contributions come from very experienced practitioners in the UK insurance industry. The other contributors are academics, but from a wider than usual range of disciplines. There are lawyers, business academics, philosophers, and one political theorist. There is also a contribution prepared by scientists in the UK Medical Research Council. This piece reflects the bearing of genetics research on insurance practice. All the contributors work in Britain, and are at home both theoretically and practically with the existence here of a large welfare state. So some of the economic and social assumptions of the American literature are absent in what follows.

The book is divided into two parts. In the first part, the contributors concentrate on ethical issues in private sector health, life and related forms of insurance. These issues are to do with (1) the fairness of access to the insurance market; (2) the fairness of charges to those who have access but who belong to groups at high risk of an insured loss; and (3) conflicts between what is necessary for risk assessment (underwriting) in a profitable insurance industry and different individual rights – ranging from a right to privacy to a possible right of remaining in ignorance of disturbing medical information. In the second part, contributors turn to the ethics of public health insurance, and the ethical values reflected in an increased role for private provision for hospital care, long-term care and income support.

PART I: THE ETHICS OF UNDERWRITING

The organisation of Part I caters for different types of reader. There are articles for those who are concerned with the ethical issues surrounding insurance for AIDS sufferers, for those who have conditions for which there are or may in the future be genetic tests, for the disabled. There are also articles for those who want an overview of the ethics of underwriting – whether on its own, or as a supplement to the discussions of the more particular issues.

Overview articles

The overview articles take the form of a spirited argument for the freedom to underwrite – put by a prominent UK underwriter, Spencer Leigh – and a mildly disagreeing response from myself. Spencer Leigh's article is based on an award-winning and controversial long article presented to working members of the Institute of Actuaries in London in January 1996. Leigh argues that claims of unfair insurers' discrimination against AIDS sufferers or those with genetic diseases do not come to grips with the rationale of underwriting. Underwriting or risk assessment, along with other insurance conventions, is justified by the principle that insurers have a right to know what risks they are taking on before accepting them. There is enormous scope for concealing from insurers the risk that an insurance applicant knows he has of falling ill or dying or suffering some other loss. And there has to be some countervailing scope for refusing insurance applications from some people, or disputing claims when misrepresentation has led to an underestimate of risk. The convention of maximum good faith in British insurance, according to which the obligation is on the insured to inform the insurer of any fact or change of circumstances that affects the risks under an insurance policy is justified in the same way. So are the lifestyle questions put to young single men who apply for high life cover. So might be the request for the results of genetic tests.

My reply to Leigh is an argument to the conclusion that the freedom to underwrite is limited. The worse the consequences for the uninsured of being refused insurance, the less morally justified the refusal. But this consequentialist argument does not necessarily show that *private* insurers have to take on some bad risks. The conclusion is probably that it is immoral not to have a comprehensive, *public* insurance scheme – at any rate for medical insurance. Underwriting for medical insurance beyond that provided through a public scheme may be justified. So may underwriting for commercial life insurance, especially if the amount of cover is very large. But it is consistent with this that, for relatively low payouts, insurance should be available on standard terms to everyone, perhaps without much investigation of the risks carried by applicants. Again, where policies are for large sums, a certain amount of intrusive questioning to establish risk may be justified that would not be justified for smaller policies. The ethics of private health insurance require scruples in insurers about the quality of the evidence they use to assess risk and scruples in insurance applicants about honesty in applications. The ethics of *public* health insurance require more of everyone: more of the individuals who pay and more of the individuals who receive cover without being able to pay. More is required, because the ethics of public insurance are the ethics of solidarity with other insured people, and with health care workers, whose services may be only modestly recompensed by a public scheme, and whose advice is often ignored by those who might benefit from it.

Articles on specific issues

Should every scientific finding and method that assists in the assessment of insurance risk be available to private insurers? The question is given a particular edge by on-going international research programmes in genetics that promise genetic tests for a whole range of diseases and disabilities and which may suggest associations between different genetic profiles and predispositions to crime, violence or other traits which insurers, employers and others may want to exploit. Many ethical problems surround the pursuit and application of genetics research, quite apart from issues connected with insurance. Both the science and some of the ethical questions recognised by investigators are reviewed systematically in Chapter 3.

Chapter 4 takes up the consequences of genetics research for insurance in particular. McLean and Gannon think that issues of confidentiality and privacy are crucial. How much are insurers entitled to find out about insurance applicants, given that, in the UK at any rate, their risks are reduced by the law governing insurance contracts, which puts the burden on insurance applicants and policyholders to disclose everything they know about themselves and their circumstances that increases the risk being insured against. Risks are further reduced by information about the medical history of policyholders and applicants and their families. Is it reasonable to

4

reduce the risks of insurers further by making the approval of insurance applications depend on compulsory genetic testing? McLean and Gannon have doubts. In addition to the general ethical presumption against coercion, there is the fact that genetic tests often disclose things that are upsetting to find out and sometimes difficult to take medical measures against. Perhaps patients have the right to refuse tests in these circumstances, and perhaps insurers have no right to require tests. Patients have an even stronger ground for refusal where the results of tests are open to more than one interpretation, and where there is a good chance that cautious insurers will assume the worst and refuse an application or load the premiums heavily.

The question of using genetic tests in underwriting is similar to the question of using HIV tests in underwriting. Finding out that one is HIV positive is often a catastrophe, and until recently the information would have led automatically to the refusal of private health or life insurance. In jurisdictions where disclosure of medical information is not compulsory, and where the 'utmost good faith' convention of British insurance does not apply, people have managed to get very large insurance pay-outs by lying in their applications. On the other hand, some people without HIV disease have been charged disproportionate amounts for insurance for no other reason than that they have been disputably classified by insurers as high-risk. A regime of testing acts against both applicant fraud and insurer prejudice, but making a test compulsory has some of the drawbacks pointed out in Chapter 4. Since the early 1990s British insurers have asked applicants whether they have had AIDS tests, but the practice of refusing insurance or loading premiums for those who have taken tests has apparently died out. Lifestyle questionnaires have got more explicit, however. Have they invaded the privacy of insurance applicants? Not necessarily, according to Chapter 5. Draper argues that straight questions and answers may be better than unjust jumping to conclusions. The reasonableness of intrusiveness and of refusal of applications rises with the amount of cover applied for, especially in places where private insurers operate alongside a comprehensive public health service. She takes account of innovating American insurance practice – which extends cover – at a price – even to the HIV positive, and she calls attention to the unreasonableness of catastrophic illness cover for those at risk as health care workers of contracting HIV disease.

The disabled have been perceived by the insurance industry as higher-risk applicants for a whole range of insurance – even household and motor insurance. Recent legislation makes the loading of premiums in this way illegal unless it is based on medical evidence. A clear change for the better, one would have thought. Chapter 6 shows how morally motivated legislation improves the lot of the disabled in theory, but in practice increases the costs of insurers, who have to pay to produce data on the risks carried by various kinds of disability. As in the cases considered by Chapters 4 and 5, insurers have a choice. They can relax their assessment of risk and charge non-discriminatory standard rates to disabled and non-disabled alike, in which case they can expect to make more pay-outs than necessary; or they can check zealously for evidence of increased risk, which is itself costly and may invite legal action. The requirements of the insurance market and the purpose of the new anti-discrimination legislation may in the end cancel one another out.

PART II: PUBLIC OR PRIVATE PROVISION?

Part II broaches the biggest question now facing the welfare state in Western Europe. How can the rising cost of care and rising expectations among the public be reconciled with the need for balanced public spending and the moral requirement that all those who need care should have reasonable access to it? 'Care' here covers not only hospital care for those with acute illness but also the whole range of services in long-stay facilities for the elderly or the mentally ill, for children in care, for the disabled, and so on.

In Chapter 7 Albert Weale considers whether it is really possible in practice for a health service to live up simultaneously to the three ideals of health care provision in the welfare state: that it should be comprehensive in the range of health care it delivers, that it should be high-quality, and that it should be available to all who need it. These ideals are probably *not* simultaneously realisable; but then, neither is it possible to get out of the difficulty by dropping one of the ideals. All the most commonly canvassed ways out – reducing the comprehensiveness and allowing some treatment to be available only through private insurance; giving priority of treatment to certain conditions or certain types of patient; or maintaining comprehensiveness and universal availability but at the cost of treating everyone less effectively and after a longer and longer wait – are open to telling objections. And the pattern of unsatisfactory and ineliminatable trade-offs is as inescapable in health as in other areas of public policy. The governing ideals in these different areas are individually legitimate *and* jointly in tension.

Chapter 8 considers in more detail the way that private medical insurance can complement public health care provision. Private medical insurance can not only introduce extra money for health care without adding to public spending totals, it can introduce disciplines that make treatments more effective without being more expensive; it can introduce disincentives to the misuse of primary care facilities. And it can do all these things without necessarily alienating users of a public sector health service. These are the conclusions reached by David Cavers, who headed Norwich Union Healthcare until his untimely death while this volume was in preparation. David was working on revisions of his chapter until he succumbed to a long illness, and this volume is dedicated to him and his willingness to try to build bridges between ethicists and the insurance industry.

Chapter 9 is a sustained account of the good that defenders of public insurance want to protect and claim is threatened by any move in the direction of private insurance: equality of access to health care. Cartwright shows how it is easy to read inequality of access into many sets of circumstances that do not impugn the justice of a given system of health care distribution, and he shows how the morally important kind of equality of access to health care depends on a certain philosophical conception of persons. He goes on to claim that certain choices of the treatments to make available through a public health service do not fit in with this conception of persons. He takes issue with the standards of equality of access implicit in Weale and Cavers.

The last two chapters take up the relative merits of public and private provision in the light of the whole range of care that the welfare state has traditionally provided, not all of it narrowly medical. They ask how changes in the birth rate, increased longevity and high expectations can produce a population big enough and rich enough to fund pensions, long-term care and other things from taxation alone. In Chapter 10 Booth and Dickinson argue that private sector insurance solutions are both economically desirable and morally defensible. Part of the moral argument is to do with considerations of generational justice: far from encouraging solidarity between generations, social insurance arrangements can lead to conflict between them, because the later generation inherits the burdens of caring for their elders without necessarily having the means of meeting them.

In Chapter 11 Peter Moore considers the evolution in the UK of insurance involvement in pensions. Developments in the financial services industry around the world have forced insurers to enter markets that they have traditionally left to others, at times with unfortunate results. The relatively recent marketing of pensions in the UK has left many people worse off than they otherwise would have been, while longer-standing problems in private pension provision have not entirely been overcome. The precarious access of divorced women to pension benefits is a case in point. Despite these problems, insurance companies are bound to have an increasingly big role in the provision of pensions. Public sector pension schemes around the world are hugely overextended financially, and will become intolerably overextended in the future. For similar reasons, public provision of long-term care for the elderly may come to be unaffordable without the involvement of the insurance industry.

NOTE

1 See Nancy Kass, 'Insurance for the insurers: the use of genetic tests', *Hastings Center Report* 22, 6 (1992), pp. 6–11; Thomas Murray, 'The moral mission of health insurance', *Hastings Center Report* 22, 6 (1992), pp. 12–17. For a broader view see 'Use of genetic data, employment and insurance: an international perspective', *Bioethics* 7, 2–3 (1993), pp. 126–34.

Part I

THE ETHICS OF
UNDERWRITING

1

THE FREEDOM TO UNDERWRITE

Spencer Leigh

In the commercial world, an essential requirement of completing a contract is an agreement between the parties as to its nature and scope. Each person is deemed to be equally able to assess the value of the bargain offered. Hence the maxim 'let the buyer beware' (*caveat emptor*). This does not apply to life assurance, as the proposer may know more about himself than the insurer could possibly discover. The information could relate to health, habits, occupation, family history and financial standing. Therefore the law imposes on the proposer the duty of 'utmost good faith' (*uberrima fides*). In my view, only a fool or a rogue would disagree with this principle. Furthermore, the risk selection procedures used by life offices have been accepted by doctors and by the public for many years. Nevertheless, various groups want us to make concessions for social and medical reasons. The rights of the individual are being championed everywhere, and so it is unrealistic for offices to hope for Freedom to Underwrite as we approach the year 2000. Who is right – the critics, or the industry?

For a peaceful life, the easiest option is for insurers to give in to the critics. However, that could cost the industry dear. As I hope to demonstrate, the Freedom to Underwrite is not something to relinquish lightly. The Freedom to Underwrite is being eroded as a result of AIDS lobby groups, regulations regarding genetic testing and legislation over disability. And who knows what else is around the corner? In what follows I try to be objective, but I know that my training disposes me to side with the insurers.[1]

DEFINING THE FREEDOM TO UNDERWRITE

Until the mid-1980s the general public paid no attention to life underwriting. Since the advent of AIDS, life underwriters have come under the spotlight. We have become the subject of newspaper editorials, and there was even a private member's Bill to limit our powers in 1994! We should be proud that we have such a high profile but we must be sure that we can defend our position.

Many of the issues raised by the question of the Freedom to Underwrite are easy to see from two sides. Usually they involve drawing the line between equity and equality, and – let's face it – life assurance underwriting is about discrimination, although we call it 'selection'. 'Discrimination' is a word with very negative connotations today, but a distinction should be drawn between fair and unfair discrimination. Fair discrimination is where a proposer's risk has been properly evaluated and is reflected in the premiums. Unfair discrimination is when equal risks are not treated equally. Such action is always unreasonable but fair discrimination is essential to good underwriting practice. A life office should strive for an unbiased assessment of the risk. It is sound business practice that the premiums charged should relate to the risk an individual brings to the fund.

In the early 1980s, before the advent of AIDS, there was total freedom to underwrite. A life office could do what it wanted, and this was manifest in three ways:

- *Proposals.* On its proposal forms, a life office could ask whatever it considered relevant. Up to the mid-1960s, offices asked proposers about their ethnic origins and even charged so-called racial extras. They based them on such facts as an Indian's expectation of life being less than an Englishman's, although no one had figures for Indians living in England. Following the Race Relations Act 1968, offices removed the additional premiums from existing contracts and resolved not to charge them for new proposals. It was a minor infringement of the Freedom to Underwrite at the time, but I doubt if the extras were needed in the first place.
- *Medical evidence.* An underwriter could request whatever medical evidence he thought was necessary, usually a report from the GP (a medical attendant's report or MAR) or a medical examination report (MER). Again, there were no restrictions regarding the questions on those forms.
- *Underwriting decision.* An underwriter could make whatever decision he thought was appropriate – ordinary rates, a rating, postponement of cover or outright declinature.

In various ways, there have been challenges to:

- The questions on proposals and supplementary forms.
- The questions on MARs.
- The questions on MERs.
- The decisions made by underwriters.
- The exclusion clauses put on policies.

As will be seen, the AIDS lobby has won one victory, admittedly not a substantial one, and many interested parties are attacking the Freedom to Underwrite. In the climate of the late-1990s, with sympathy for the rights of the individual at an all-time high, life offices could alienate many of the public by demanding the Freedom to Underwrite. Even if they believe they have right on their side, they have to be very careful about how they present their arguments.

The various threats to the Freedom to Underwrite are not exclusive to the UK and they have been raised with different emphases and different outcomes in many other countries. However, comparison between one country and the UK can be made only after considering all the relevant facts, as the provision of insurance, existing legislation and medical practice can vary considerably. Thanks to the National Health Service, everyone in the UK is assigned to a GP and, as a result, we are able to request MARs, a facility that exists in few other countries. In the US it is common practice to use private investigators to check out claims for non-disclosure: in the UK they tend only to be used in connection with the more dramatic potential frauds.

Pressure groups, however, may take the most favourable solution from thirty or forty countries and display it as a model. I may sound xenophobic, but Great Britain is a major player on the world stage in insurance, and I find it odd that we should be asked to follow countries that we would not dream of following in anything else. Even following the US has its problems, and a cautious note was added by Dr Robert Pokorski, the Chief Medical Officer of North American Reassurance/Swiss Re in the US and an important voice of the industry in the debate on genetic testing. When talking to UK life underwriters early in 1995, he said, 'Everybody follows us and the danger is that we are going to do something really stupid.' Ultimately, however, it must be recognised that the UK may be affected by legislation from the EU.

AIDS

The advent of AIDS in the mid-1980s caused new problems for life offices. Not only did they have to consider what action to take; they had to consider what criticism they might receive from AIDS pressure groups. From the start, there was criticism of the questions on the proposal which asked applicants to disclose details of previous HIV tests and whether they had been counselled for HIV. The wording that offices followed in the early 1990s was along these lines:

- Have you ever been personally counselled or medically advised in connection with AIDS or sexually transmitted diseases?
- Have you ever had an HIV/AIDS test? If so, please give details, dates and results.

The word 'personally' was included at the request of the AIDS pressure group, the Terrance Higgins Trust. They argued that everyone in the UK had been counselled for HIV by having leaflets through their letter boxes and so would have to answer 'Yes'. Strictly speaking they may have been right, but the criticism smacked of their desperation at the sight of any questions about HIV status on insurance proposals.

The question itself identified those who were HIV positive, if they told the truth, and it also helped to identify those who were at high risk. In essence, if someone was having regular HIV tests, he or she might be following a life style which could lead to AIDS. An office might request a medical examination and its own HIV test in such cases. There was a difference of emphasis here, as the Terrance Higgins Trust thought that regular HIV testing was more a sign of social responsibility than of promiscuity.

It is hard to avoid emotive language, but someone may have an HIV test for entirely 'innocent' reasons. To cover this, life offices added the words: 'To enable us to process your application as quickly as possible, please indicate whether the test was for routine screening (e.g. blood donation, antenatal, employment) or for any other reason and give details, including the date and the result.' If, for example, a female said she had an AIDS test during pregnancy and the result was negative, the underwriter would disregard the information.

In the early days of AIDS, one office declined two proposers who had had HIV tests, solely on the grounds that they had had a test.

This mistake cost the industry dear, as the view was formed that life offices were refusing cover to all those who had had HIV tests. This led to the ABI stating that individuals would not be refused cover or charged more *solely* on the basis of negative HIV tests.

That is true. I know that my own office has never refused anyone life insurance *solely* as a result of previous HIV tests. Why should we? It does not make sense, as we want to accept as much business as practicable. However, the question may reveal someone who is at high risk from AIDS. As a spokesman for Commercial Union bravely put it, 'The vast majority of people who go for a test do so because they feel they have put themselves at risk in some way. If they are liable to engage in high risk activities, then we believe that it should be taken into consideration.'

The question about the AIDS risk was sensible and businesslike, but the public continues to dislike it. Some doctors, AIDS lobby groups, led by the Terrance Higgins Trust, and the Consumers' Association argued for a change to the question. The curious view was formed that some people who were at risk might decide against an HIV test because they might want life assurance in the future and would thus have to declare it on a proposal. It seemed to me that they were all complaining on behalf of somebody else, because in all the years that the issue was raised I never came across anyone to whom this applied. Besides, it is always possible to have an HIV test anonymously and, at the time of a claim, a life office could never establish that the proposer knew he was HIV positive.

The unlikeliness of their complaint can be seen when it is taken out of the AIDS arena. You could not imagine anyone saying, 'I've got chest pains, but I won't have an ECG because I may have to declare it on a life assurance proposal in the future.' The public thinks very little about insurance.

Nevertheless, it was considered that the attitude of insurance companies to those who had undergone an HIV test had been a deterrent to people taking tests in the first place. The ABI disputed this and in 1991 they jointly sponsored a survey with the Department of Health. The report, *AIDS and Life Insurance*, was published by HMSO and it concluded that 'it is definitely the case that there are some people who are put off taking an HIV test because of the questions on insurance proposal forms'. I would not disagree with that – there must be *some* people, however misguided, and maybe only a few, who would be put off having an HIV test for this reason.

The report commented on the size of the problem, 'We are confident that in percentage terms it will be very small, probably considerably less than 1 per cent.' This was good news for the industry – effectively, the proposal questions made no difference to the decisions of over 99 per cent of the population. However, in gross numbers 'it would certainly be in the thousands, possibly in the tens of thousands'.

That final remark undid the good work of the survey. Virginia Bottomley, then Minister of Health, described the results as 'worrying' and said that such questions could be hindering the government's attempts to halt the spread of AIDS. The newspapers, with a disregard for numeracy, ran headlines like 'AIDS questions puts off thousands'. The trade press, which should at least have been supportive, ran negative stories: the industry was shooting itself in the foot, and an onslaught on the AIDS question was inevitable. The Terrance Higgins Trust referred to the 'disgraceful practice' and *The Times* (13 November 1993) said, 'Many people have been discouraged from taking an HIV test for fear that, irrespective of the result, it will disqualify them from obtaining life insurance.' It appeared that the big bad insurance companies were making unreasonable requests of their clients.

In 1994 Lord Jellicoe introduced a private member's Bill in Parliament which would have compelled insurance companies to change their ways. The question would simply ask a proposer whether he or she was HIV positive. If the Bill were to be debated in the House, the situation could be grim for the industry. Consider how the provisions of the Criminal Justice Bill, also a private member's Bill, were amended on the floor of the House. Who could say what amendments would be tabled, and, in view of various insurance scandals, the industry was short of politcial friends. Any MP who said, 'The industry is doing a good job and no legislation is necessary', would have been howled down.

Parliamentary time is always at a premium and Ministers are always wanting to reduce the agenda. Therefore the Department of Health discussed Lord Jellicoe's Bill with the ABI to see whether some quasi-legislation could be agreed. From January 1995 the ABI recommended to offices that proposals should not request details of HIV/AIDS tests unless the result was positive. In effect, this was quasi-legislation, and the revised question was:

> Have you ever been tested positive for HIV/AIDS or Hepatitis B or C, or have you been tested/treated for other sexually transmitted diseases, or are you awaiting the result of such a test?

All members accepted the position. Personally, I felt the question was convoluted and I did not see the purpose of bringing Hepatitis B or C into the equation.

The Times (15 December 1994) was delighted. In an editorial it stated,

> In many beneficial respects, the deterrents to testing for HIV are at last being reduced. Primary amongst them used to be the insurance companies' attitudes to those who had undergone a test, whatever the result. To discriminate against the socially responsible was as insulting as it was counter-productive. Now, after years of pressure, the insurers have agreed to ask only whether an applicant has been tested positive.

A little of the Freedom to Underwrite had been lost. Offices could no longer find out whether someone had had regular HIV tests. On the other hand, in the media there was nothing but praise for the change.

During the course of the debate I heard two highly individualistic ways of determining a suitable question, neither of which, I am sure, would have been acceptable. One was 'Are there any factors in your life which might put you at risk of HIV infection?' This is too subjective: someone could be having the time of his life every night and yet believe, quite erroneously, that he was not putting himself at risk – e.g. AIDS happens to older men. Hence the question could be answered honestly, 'No'. Similarly, I have heard it suggested that an office should ask, 'Are you prepared to take an HIV test?' This was a gloriously Catch-22 question. Anyone who answers 'No' should be asked to go for one.

If you score a point you try again, and so the change on proposal forms is not going to be the end of the matter. Ivan Massow, an independent financial adviser whose company specialises in gay clients, wrote in *Financial Adviser* (9 February 1995): 'When I opened an office in Edinburgh, the city seemed a monument to pompous, self-righteous propriety that housed some of the most vindictive life assurance underwriters. They sat in their emerald castles and passed judgment on the promiscuous behaviour of homosexual men.' One of Ivan Massow's arguments is that the industry does not know what it is doing. The Government Actuary has told offices that the recommended projection of AIDS deaths contained some safety margin. Ivan Massow said in *Money Marketing*: 'It would seem that everything that its smug underwriters have predicted has turned out to be totally incorrect.' Going by my own experience, only a handful of proposers have ever complained about the AIDS question on proposals, but several have objected to the life-style questionnaire. This is a series of questions relating to the sexual orientation of a proposer and his or her partners, and it could be that those who complain have most to gain by not complet-ing it. As a result of this, a homosexual in a stable relationship with a negative HIV test is likely to be charged an extra premium of around £3 per annum for each £1,000 sum assured.

Surprisingly, there has not been wholesale criticism of the HIV test itself, provided that there has been proper counselling. Occasionally policyholders refuse to have an HIV test, but they usually relent. I was surprised when the Terrance Higgins Trust even suggested a lowering of the automatic HIV test limits as a trade-off for a change in the question.

The AIDS debate has occasionally gone outside its boundaries and shown the direction that industry criticism is going. Baroness Gardner of Parkes in the House of Lords (1 December 1994) said,

> On health grounds, I think it wrong that anyone should ask whether a patient has had any negative test of any type, whether it is a test for breast screening, or a chest X-ray or any other sort of test. Surely it must be good that a person should be screened for a condition rather than have that held against him when applying for insurance.

This is a misguided view, because the underlying reason for the test is surely important, and the negative test may not guarantee there is no disease. Taking it to the limit, we might end up with just one ques-tion, 'Are you healthy?', and if you answer 'Yes', you can have cover at standard rates.[2]

GENETICS – THE BACKGROUND

Genetic testing can predict a person's future health. Genes pass characteristics from parents to their children, and the information is stored in the molecule DNA (deoxyribonucleic acid). A complete set of genes is in each of the body's cells, irrespective of their particular purpose. As there may be over 50,000 in our bodies and only 10 per cent have been identified in terms of an inherited characteristic or disease, an enormous amount of research remains to be done. Having said that, developments have been swift, particularly in the US, and any timetable is likely to be brought forward. It is possible that all the genes in our bodies will have been identified by the year 2000.

Genes are unaltered throughout life, so the results of a test will be the same no matter when it is performed. Genetic testing of children is controversial because a child is not old enough to give its consent and, in later years, may not want to have had such knowledge. Conversely, the parents' authority is surely valid if some preventative measures can be taken straightaway. Even more contentious is pre-natal testing, which may lead to questions of abortion.

Some abnormalities are so significant that the disease is certain to manifest itself in everyone so identified. These monogenic disorders are caused by a single defect, but fortunately they are rare. However, there are many more common diseases for which multi-factorial genetic tests indicate susceptibility. These polygenic disorders include cancer and heart disease.

Huntington's chorea is a slow, wasting disease in which the patient's progressive mental and physical disability leads to involuntary movements, dementia and then premature death. Huntington's chorea is still incurable, and if someone is carrying the gene, he will get the disease, although he may not have the symptoms until he is fifty. It is a rare disease – even the quoted figure of 1 in 10,000 seems excessive – and the most noted sufferer was the American folk singer Woody Guthrie. In the past, a proposer with a family history of Huntington's chorea would be refused life assurance or given a high additional premium, even though no symptoms might be present. This was because the life office could not know whether a proposer would succumb to the disease – and there was a 50 per cent chance of it happening. Now it is possible for someone to be tested for the disorder; the tests are almost 100 per cent accurate, and becoming more so as the months go by.

Genetic tests are also available for other inherited fatal diseases such as muscular dystrophy, cystic fibrosis, polycystic kidneys and Marfan's syndrome. So, effectively, many people who would have been denied insurance should now be able to obtain it – provided there is evidence of a negative test. These diseases are not regularly encountered by life underwriters although, taken together, they are significant. However, life offices have long been interested in inherited diseases. Why else are questions about family history asked on proposals? A history of heart disease in both parents may give rise to a medical examination and, perhaps, an additional premium. As has often been said, the surest way to a long life is to choose your parents carefully.

Genetic testing will be significant for the most common disorders because it can determine a predisposition towards heart disease, certain types of cancer, and many other complaints. Here the situation is very different from Huntington's chorea. If you have a positive genetic test for Huntington's chorea, you will develop the disease. If you have a positive genetic test for heart disease, you may develop the disease but the genes are just one of several factors, including smoking, eating, stress and lack of exercise. Indeed, someone with a positive test for heart disease may take measures to reduce the risk by changing his life style. Again, someone with a positive test for cancer may receive regular screening so that an early diagnosis can be made and treatment given. Tests may also be developed for predispositions to other genetic disorders such as Alzheimer's disease, asthma, diabetes, epilepsy, high blood pressure, mental illness and even alcoholism.

The science of applying such genetic tests will take years to develop but, although the results may be open to interpretation, they will become a fact of life. Initially, those with significant family histories may be tested, but in twenty years, perhaps, the tests may be available to everyone. It would not surprise me if Westerners carried round a smartcard containing their genetic profile. From a life assurance viewpoint, this could lead to a no-win situation – people with perfect genes would want insurance only against accidents and infectious diseases, and the rest would not be prepared to pay the extra premiums.

Even more mind-boggling is genetic engineering, which can correct genetic disorders. Some gene transplants have already taken place in the US and the process may be no more disagreeable than a blood transfusion. This is all very well for treating disease but there are ethical and religious problems if a change is requested for non-medical reasons: for example, someone might want to become a better athlete or change the colour of his or her skin. The common good of allowing people to be as they want to be has to be measured against potential abuses and, of course, some would argue that it is always best for people to stick with the genes with which they were born. But then again, who is to say that the genes of embryos will not also be changed?

All this is in the future, but that future is not far away. The first genetically related insurance policy has already been developed by a Lloyd's syndicate. A policy, which can be effected by a pregnant mother, provides a payment if a child is born with one of five genetic disorders.

What does a life office do now about genetic testing? A proposal asks the client in general terms about medical tests and, all things being equal, those should include genetic tests. A proposer who withholds the information is withholding material facts. In years to come, when the tests are more common, they may be specifically referred to on the proposal. A typical question might be 'Have you ever had a test to see whether you have inherited the gene for any disease? If so, please give the reason and the result.' There is no point in putting such a question on today's forms, as it would confuse most clients. Even with the consent of the proposer, it may be difficult for a third party such as a life office to obtain written confirmation of the results. A life office that is not able to obtain confirmation will have to decide each case on its merits.

The last few years have seen the development of preferred lives insurance. Here proposers qualify for a discount of around 15 per cent if they do not smoke, have a good family history, a good medical and no other specified risk factors. This is said to be cherry-picking, although the term has unfortunate negative connotations. The offices concerned have stressed that it is not connected with genetic testing. Not at the moment, that is. It is possible that preferred life insurance will become the norm, and that different criteria will be used to assess preferred lives. However, 'Genetic testing ABI Code of Practice' states that 'insurers might not offer individuals lower than standard premiums on the basis of Genetic Test results'.

It has been suggested that life offices should show an enlightened view and specifically state that proposers need not give details of genetic testing. In other words, for whatever good reason, they should be allowed to lie. To date, few people have had genetic tests, but a life office naturally wants to know the results. The underlying concept of insurance is that proposers pay for the risks they bring to the fund, and if a life office does not seek the information, it may be selected against by clients who are privy to certain information about themselves. A client with a positive genetic test for heart disease might be tempted to propose for critical illness policies with several offices. Recently, some old samples of the US politician Hubert Humphrey have been tested. It has been discovered that his bladder cancer could have been diagnosed with genetic testing over ten years before he had any symptoms. Think of the damage individuals could inflict on the industry with similar knowledge about themselves. In short, if the proposer knows the results of genetic testing, then the life office wants to know them too. Problems obviously arise if tests can be taken anonymously, as no one is able to establish what is known at the time of proposing, just as with HIV testing.

Are life offices likely to ask proposers to undergo genetic testing? Not in the short term, and no movement is likely until such time as the tests have been fully accepted and endorsed by the medical fraternity. Even then, life offices are unlikely to recommend testing until the principle has been accepted by the general public. In short, life offices are loathe to initiate social change but they have to respond to it. If genetic tests can be taken privately, then I think the results will be wanted by insurance companies, and they will want the right to test individuals. If genetic tests become a regular and acceptable routine that people regard as part of a regular health check, they could become part of the underwriting process. If not, it is unlikely that underwriters will call for genetic testing except to clarify the position on a person with an already identified problem. And think of the people who have favourable genetic tests. Would they not want to use the information to obtain standard terms, or even to request a discount? It is often overlooked that many proposers would benefit from genetic testing. They might object strongly to not being allowed to use the information to obtain more favourable rates. Those with a good genetic profile may create a run on the annuity market, so should we be asking medical questions there as well? Again, those with an unfavourable genetic profile could be given increased rates.

Research laboratories may be unwilling to undertake testing for insurance companies, but once the testing can be done commercially, the laboratories will be actively encouraging offices to use them. It is inevitable, because commercial organisations will wish to test as many people as possible, thereby ensuring a reduction in unit costs. Life offices are unlikely to request tests for all individuals but it may become obligatory for the larger proposals (£1 million or more), and for smaller proposals with a significant family history. The test itself will present few problems and should be no more difficult to arrange than tests for blood sugar or cholesterol, and there are no physical risks to the proposer. The cost may be high, but one national newspaper has reported that tests will become available for a mere £2. Such economies of scale are likely only if the whole UK population is screened. The main problem, as with HIV testing, will relate to counselling both before and after the test so that clients are fully aware of its nature. The counselling may need to be extensive and may have to involve the proposer's family. There have been patronising comments in the press that individuals cannot properly consent to these tests because they do not appreciate what they are authorising in the first place. But there is every reason to think that appropriate counselling will resolve this.

Another problem occurs with those who do not wish to know their genetic profile. Their way of life may be changed by a positive diagnosis and they may prefer to remain ignorant. But this could apply to anyone who attends a medical examination for life assurance – and there is no counselling there. When a life office feels that genetic information is necessary, the office may have to say, 'Sorry, but we can't give you the cover you require without this test.'

Life offices currently accept 95 per cent of all proposals on standard terms. However, about one in ten of all genetic screenings for heart disease will be positive. Should a life office increase the premium for that alone? This is uncharted territory, but it could lead to a totally new concept in life assurance – there might be less grouping via standard rates and instead each proposer would be individually assessed and a process akin to motor or household insurance would take place. However, at this point in time, life offices do not want a small healthy pool: they want to offer cover to as many clients as possible.

The whole question as to whether insurance companies should be allowed to use genetic information is controversial. In California legislation was being introduced which would have allowed an individual to conceal information about genetic testing from a life office but extensive lobbying by the industry was successful and the proposed legislation was vetoed by the Governor. A ban on genetic screening as a condition of an insurance policy has been recommended to the European Parliament. The recommendation, made in 1992, said, 'Insurers should not have the right to require genetic testing or to enquire about the results of previously performed tests as a precondition for the conclusion or modification of an insurance contract.'

Once again, it appears that insurance principles are not understood by the industry's critics, although it is possible that the insurance companies decided that the financial risk was not too great and so withheld their lobbying. However, a ban on genetic screening could leave insurance companies and their funds unprotected. Life offices have to protect themselves from proposers who know the results of genetic or other tests which reveal a poor outlook. It is reasonable to ask proposers about all the tests they have previously undergone, including genetic ones.

The Health Council of the Netherlands has stated, 'We find it unacceptable that people affected from birth with a genetic predisposition should be faced with additional social obstacles, and that their relatives should also be at a disadvantage in this way.' That is a total misunderstanding of the principles of insurance.

The current trend is to argue that someone who contracts a serious disease through no fault of their own should not be penalised. This way of thinking reflects real concern and is very understandable. Consider the views of Professor Bob Williamson, a geneticist from St Mary's Hospital Medical School in London. He draws a distinction between information over which people have no control (genes) and factors which are matters of choice (smoking, sports). He has called for legislation so that 'the former is not used to discriminate against individuals'. In other words, we should impose an extra premium when it is the proposer's own fault; otherwise, we are being unfair. It is not the life offices that are being unfair, but life itself. In any event, for most purposes, differential rates are used for males and females, surely something over which a person has no control. Quite simply, if a proposer is more likely than the average person of the same sex and the same age to die prematurely, the premium should be higher: it is the increased probability of death that is important to the life office and not how it has arisen.[3]

Another angle for the industry relates to employment medicals. Some hapless individuals may find it difficult to gain employment because the results of their genetic tests suggest higher levels of sickness in the future. Similarly, with on-going medical checks, some of the existing work force may be dismissed for the same reason. The tabloids will have a field day with headlines like 'My genes got me the sack'. The question of employment is particularly pertinent in the US. There is no equivalent of the NHS, and so employers may be liable to provide health care benefits to an employee and his family. Genetic tests may be requested on the family as a whole and decisions reached about the potential liability.

The issues facing the insurance industry over genetic testing are immense and, in some ways, they can be seen as a re-enactment of the issues surrounding HIV testing and AIDS. However, there are distinct differences – genetic testing can affect the entire insured population and, unlike AIDS, this cannot lead to any extra deaths. Indeed, the whole thrust of genetic testing is to improve mortality. Back to Dr Pokorski, who told UK life underwriters in 1995,

> If you thought AIDS was bad for the industry, genetics is much worse. Bad legislation has the opportunity to devastate the industry. There has to be a level playing-field between what the assured knows and what the assurer knows. We are going into unchartered territory if we change this.

In the US, the medical director of Lincoln National Life has said, 'From an underwriting point of view, insurers may wish that genetic tests had not been developed.' I don't accept this. The benefits have to be considered alongside the drawbacks, and such a negative response is as one-sided as the life offices' critics. It has never been possible to pinpoint individuals with such accuracy before and anything which enables an underwriter to make a more accurate assessment of a future risk can only be beneficial to society as a whole and to the industry.

GENETICS – THE WAY FORWARD

From the 1995 House of Commons Science and Technology Committee report *Human Science: Genetics and its Consequences*:

247. We cannot see into the future; it may be that the ABI is correct, and that the use of genetic information in insurance is limited, and raises no new problems. However, the great majority of our witnesses, including those with expertise in genetics, think that such information could have major implications for the industry in a relatively short time. In our view the ABI has reacted to these predictions with undue complacency; it would, at least, be prudent to have contingency plans in place to ensure that changes were dealt with in an orderly manner.

248. Such plans may now be being made. When we met the ABI we were told that the industry hoped to make its own proposals for dealing with genetic tests in 1995. *The Committee recommends that the insurance industry be allowed*

one year in which to propose a solution acceptable to Parlia-
ment, and that if it fails to do so a solution should be sought,
by legislation if necessary. [Emphasis in original]

It would have been possible to ignore the select committee's
recommendation in paragraph 248, to call their bluff, as it were,
and risk legislation. The ABI might have argued, for example, that
it represented profit-making organisations and why should they be
forced to make changes that will affect their profitability? That
would be foolhardy. The offices would lose goodwill and it is
likely that the legislation would be enacted and be more stringent
than any recommended solution. Self-regulation is preferable to
legislation. We would have no control over proposed legislation
once it was being discussed in the House, and the results could be
damaging to the industry. It is also easier and quicker to amend
regulations than legislation when a change is necessary.

Without any embargoes, there could be misuse of a genetic testing
by an office anxious to steal a lead over its rivals. The ABI had to
consider whether it is right to stifle competition. Certain principles
need to be addressed when considering any solution to these issues.

The principle of uberrima fides. An insurance company cannot
know everything about an individual and so it relies on the concept
of 'utmost good faith' – it can challenge a claim on the grounds of
non-disclosure. This is one of the legally accepted tenets of insurance
and it is not something we should waive lightly.

Regulations need to be reviewable, perhaps every three years. The
committee says in paragraph 247, 'We cannot see into the future'.
No one knows how genetic testing is going to develop – and nor
should we be expected to. For example, one reputable company is
already advertising a test for cystic fibrosis. The committee recommends legislation to stop testing by post and without counselling.
If this does not become law, the insurance industry has a major
problem, as clients can perform their own tests and can apply for
life insurance without anyone being aware of the results. Des Le
Grys, Managing Director of Munich Re in the UK, wrote in *The
Times*, 'The public's attitude towards genetic tests, the frequency
of genetic tests and their uses will vary with time, by country and
by group: it is not sensible to draw up rigid regulations today on
the grounds that it will always be appropriate.' Any regulations
should be reviewed over time, perhaps through a forum with the
medical profession, to reflect the changes in genetic testing.

Regulations should not involve life offices in needless expense. There is a cost to every concession. If the industry gave in to its critics, it would be involved in considerable expense. However, from the committee's report it is evident that our regulations need approval from other interested parties. A balance has to be drawn and costings made for any potential solution.

Regulations should endeavour to 'get it right first time'. There is unlikely to be a solution which will be totally acceptable to all parties. The Genetic Interest Group, for example, have radical views because they are at pains to avoid a genetic underclass. This is very commendable, but a private company such as a life office might find their requirements hard to accept. A solution should be such that pressure groups would agree not to continue with their criticism.

Regulations should be in plain English and should be comprehensible to the general public. If we tell proposers that the results of genetic testing do not have to be passed to us, we must make what we are saying precisely clear. And this is why I prefer the word 'ban' to 'moratorium'.

Regulations should cover all types of business transacted by a life office. The issues are highlighted even more with critical illness and sickness cover.

The concerns surrounding genetic testing and insurance that need to be addressed are:

Those who would benefit from genetic testing may decide otherwise because they would have to declare the test on a future proposal. Life offices cannot afford to be seen as obstructing medical progress and perhaps getting in the way of screening programmes. It is not much of a concession, at present, to say that undergoing tests does not have to be declared, provided we can retain the question about family history.

Those who do not want a genetic test may be asked to have one by a life office. Again, this is very unlikely to be an issue for some years. Perhaps in five years' time, an office might want to introduce screening for proposals over £1 million.

There may be unfair assessments of genetic information by life offices. The ABI has taken the unusual but commendable step of advertising for a genetics adviser who will provide information and presumably make recommendations. Such information can be passed to the individual life offices to discuss with their own medical officers. This should counter criticism that genetic information is going to be misinterpreted.

Life offices cannot be trusted with genetic information. Questions concerning the possible mishandling of confidential information by life offices have been raised by various geneticists. This is creating a problem when none existed. Life offices have a very good record on the confidentiality of medical information, and it seems unlikely that genetic information would go astray.

Proposed solution 1 – ban genetic testing by life offices

At present there is no danger of an insurance company requesting a genetic test on an applicant. A test for Huntington's chorea with appropriate counselling could cost £500 and no company would want to pay that. However, as the committee acknowledged, the cost of genetic testing could come down and the position could change dramatically. The cost, however, is still likely to be substantial on account of the counselling. So many issues have to be taken into consideration, not least the possibilities that someone may learn that his parents are not his biological parents and that other family members may be affected.

Dr Pokorski said that having a ban for a few years on requesting genetic tests was ill conceived, even though life offices would not be giving much away.

> It puts the boot on the wrong foot and it would be very hard to remove it when you wanted to. At this point though, it would be disastrous for offices to say that they were going to carry out their own tests – they can only follow this course when the tests become commonplace as, of course, they will. Remember too that most people are going to have favourable genes and they will want insurance companies to take that into account. The US male believes in 'every man for himself' so he wants the best terms possible – he isn't going to subsidise anyone else. You wouldn't get someone in New York paying an extra for earthquakes on his house insurance to subsidise people in California.

Proposed solution 2 – ban the questioning of clients about previous genetic tests

This may be conceded, but if a test has been done, life offices should be allowed to know the result. They would expect to be told the result of a screening for cervical cancer, so why should a genetic test be different? No questions about genetic testing appear on life assurance proposals – and at the moment there is no point in including one. Most people would be confused by the question.

Suggested code of practice – genetic testing[4]

What follows is purely a suggestion I devised after reading the committee's report. It has no official status whatsoever, but the outcome could be along these lines:

- A genetic test can determine whether an individual is susceptible to a particular inherited disease.
- At present life offices do not request genetic tests on proposers for life or sickness insurance.
- Individuals are expected to answer questions on a proposal truthfully. They should give details of any medical tests undergone, including genetic tests, and of any information requested regarding family history.
- Any adverse results of genetic tests must, therefore, be disclosed, but they will be ignored for the purposes of life assurance where the initial sum assured on death is £50,000 or below and the proposer can confirm that no other cover has been obtained through this concession. An office will, however, take both the family history and any past or current illnesses into account when assessing proposals.
- No concessions are available for any form of sickness insurance.
- The agreement will be reviewed in two years' time and holds good until then.

We may not be using some of the genetic information mentioned above for underwriting purposes, but by requesting it the industry, with co-operation between offices, will be able to gauge the extent of the problem. This will give us concrete facts when the matter is reviewed.

Once a concessionary sum assured has been determined, the life offices can never go back, and the only way is up. Whatever the amount is, others will argue that it should be twice or five times that amount. I don't think that the ABI could realistically propose less than £10,000, but the £80,000 sum assured as advocated in Norway is too generous. We are, after all, giving some proposers something for nothing. Hence my chosen figure of £50,000. Nevertheless, this suggested concession is costlier than it appears.

The committee's report gives the incidence of some inherited diseases. For Huntington's chorea the figure is 1 in 10,000. If there are 30 million adults under the age of sixty-five, the disease affects 3,000 people. If half of them already have symptoms, then 1,500 people could submit proposals for life assurance and be underwritten with the positive results of any genetic tests being ignored. Based on family history alone, they might be accepted with an additional premium of £5 per £1,000 sum assured per annum instead of being declined. Therefore the life offices are at risk for a sum assured of £75 million in respect of concessions for this disease alone. The quoted figure is 1 in 4,000 for muscular dystrophy, which would lead to a sum assured of £180 million. The total sum assured for the monogenetic diseases might be as high as £500 million. With 100 life offices, the additional exposure of each office is £5 million on average. However, with the constant talk of mergers and takeovers, the number of offices could reduce to fifty and then the exposure would average £10 million. The offices need to fund this additional liability, and, in effect, they become part of the social services. They cease to be commercial companies making solely commercial decisions, and part of the Freedom to Underwrite would be lost.

DISABILITY – THE BACKGROUND

According to the Royal Association for Disability and Rehabilitation, around 12 per cent of the total population has some form of disability. That is 6.5 million people, and even though the majority are elderly, a considerable number are of working age. It must be stressed that many disabilities have no bearing upon an insurance company's terms.

Although I personally believe that insurance companies are relatively blameless, many disabled people have suffered social injustice in recent years – sometimes owing to lack of understanding, sometimes deliberately. It is only right that legislation should be introduced to protect their rights and to determine rules for providing services and employment. This is no easy matter, as the costs can be very considerable.

Insurance is brought into the debate as disabled people may not be able to obtain insurance on the same terms as healthy lives.

In 1982 the Committee on Restrictions against Disabled Persons said:

Many disabled people find that trying to obtain insurance reveals yet another area where they are at a disadvantage. For those who have struggled to overcome physical disability, it is particularly wounding to be told that their lives are uninsurable: and doubly so where this means that they are unable to provide the protection for their families that others not so disabled would consider normal. It can also mean that they are unable to obtain a mortgage or enter into any financial contract that requires life insurance. Even where insurance cover is granted, the premium may be loaded to such an extent that it seems disproportionate to the disability, and causes additional financial hardship to those whose finances are already stretched to the limit.

Giving an example of illogical decisions, the report continued, 'Deaf people have had to pay loaded motor car insurance premiums, although no additional premiums are required from drivers with radios, telephones or cassette players in cars.' This is a recurrent theme. In October 1994 the Research Institute of Consumer Affairs – an offshoot of *Which?* – found that thirty-six out of forty-eight companies loaded premiums for certain categories of disabled drivers. The categories were arthritis, stroke, paraplegia and multiple sclerosis. The institute's director, David Yelding, said, 'The report shows that firms discriminate without evidence to justify their actions.' Any legislation is bound to have wide implications for motor and travel insurance, although I have been concentrating on life issues.

The Americans with Disabilities Act is universally applauded in the US. It mandated equal access to products, services and benefits for 50 million who qualify under the broad definitions of disabilities in the law. The financial burden imposed on the private sector was overcome because of the emotional arguments in support of the Bill. Similar legislation has been enacted in Australia and Canada, but, generally, discrimination – or selection – is allowed when it is merited by the circumstances of each case.

In the UK it is practically impossible for a private member's Bill involving substantial legislation to become law without the backing of the government. The aim of a Bill is to draw attention to an issue and hope that the government will act upon it. That was the intention of the Civil Rights (Disabled Persons) Bill 1994.

There was no prospect of the Bill becoming law, simply because of the estimated £17 billion cost to industry, commerce and government. The proposed changes in school facilities, public transport and public buildings made the Bill prohibitive, and so the government offered all help short of assistance.

In May 1995 the Bill was brought down by a large number of formalities – eighty amendments appeared in the names of five Conservative members who had taken little, if any, part in the debates. The Minister for the Disabled, Nick Scott, lost his job. The government's mishandling of the Bill gave it and its cause much more publicity than its backers could have expected.

As part of the price the government agreed to make its own proposals in the form of legislation or codes of practice. This led to the Disability Discrimination Act 1995, which was followed by the Disability Discrimination (Services and Provisions) Regulations 1996.

DISABILITY – THE LIFE OFFICE ISSUES

Premise 1 – Life offices should be allowed to distinguish between able-bodied and disabled lives when it comes to determining risks for insurance

The process of selection is one of the fundamental features of life assurance, and yet it is tempting for any government to say that life and disability insurance must be available to all without any classification of risks. The government could then make cuts in social security benefits because the public could buy life and sickness insurance without being rejected or being charged extra premiums. Actuarial theory advising against this and illustrating how insurance companies might go insolvent may go unheeded.

Insolvency *could* come about. The Civil Rights (Disabled Persons) Bill 1994, which was brought down for other reasons, effectively banned insurers from differentiating between risks. At a guess, something of the order of an additional 50 per cent in the current expenditure on death claims might be incurred if companies were not allowed to differentiate on medical grounds. Some £1.6 billion was paid out in death claims in 1992, and although this would be a large increase, the total amount paid by life offices during the year was £33 billion. The effect would be to increase premium rates substantially. Is this really what a consumer would want?

Lord Inglewood told the House of Lords in June 1995, 'The Government will not require insurance companies to charge lower premiums than the risk insured requires simply because the risk is based on the customer's disability. I am aware of no legislation in the world which would require insurance companies to do that.'

Representatives of several disability groups have remarked that there is unfair discrimination by insurers against the disabled. At one extreme, there are militant disabled person's groups who want legislation to remove every vestige of what they see as discrimination. Such views are not going to disappear overnight.

Premise 2 – Life offices are well able to underwrite the disabled fairly

In my view – and I realise this is controversial – insurance companies do not discriminate unfairly against the disabled. In fairness to all policyholders, they assess the relative risks of all proposals presented to them and charge appropriate premiums. Fairness means equal treatment for equal risks. Indeed, life offices are more competitive than ever when it comes to charging additional premiums, and more favourable terms can be obtained now than at any time in their history.

Lord Rix, speaking in the House of Lords on 15 June 1995, said,

> My contacts in the insurance industry before and since the setting up of MENCAP City Insurance Services have given me the realisation that in some instances discrimination is based not on actuarial tables or painful commercial experience, but on what I can only describe as prejudice and ignorance. It really is quite extraordinary how usually well-informed people can blunder into ill-informed decisions – though I suppose that I should not be totally surprised when the immigration rules of certain world powers have apparently been based on the assumption that Down's syndrome is a contagious disease!

I suspect that Lord Rix is generalising from a few well chosen examples. One example was discussed by a standing committee in the House of Commons in March 1994. A proposer had been asked to pay a higher life assurance premium because he had cerebral palsy. He walked with a limp, but apart from that, he did not consider that he had any disability. The office withdrew the extra premium after it had been asked to provide statistics to prove its case. An MP told the committee, 'He was being unfairly treated because the assumption being made about his life expectancy was unfair. It was not based on evidence, but on a broad assessment of the average condition of people with cerebral palsy.'

A single case like this can harm the industry. The details are repeated in the House and in the media, and the industry is made to look foolish. Life offices are accused of excessive caution, inexperience, and acting on inadequate information. Any problem would be lack of knowledge about different types of disabilities, rather than an intrinsic problem over discrimination.

OTHER CHALLENGES

This chapter has concentrated on the most pertinent challenges to the Freedom to Underwrite – AIDS, genetics and disability. There have also been challenges to the way life offices determine premiums, which in turn affects underwriting processes. For example, US insurers had to ward off a challenge that age should not be a factor in determining premium rates.

After the most obvious factor of age, sex has most bearing on the risk most people present to an insurance company. It is easy to show that a woman is likely to live around seven years longer than a man, but unisex rates are often suggested. Some countries now have unisex rates for annuities, even though, actuarially, it makes no sense. At the present time, the only lifestyle choice we can penalise wholeheartedly, without a word of complaint, is smoking. Sooner or later there is bound to be a backlash and offices will be accused of victimising smokers.

On another front, there are regular attacks from the media and pressure groups on the Association Registry, which is administered by the ABI. It was established in 1896 for offices to enter details, in coded form, of lives they rate heavily or decline. If a life then proposes to another office, the registry provides a check against possible non-disclosure. Although the criticism is unjustified, I cannot see the Association Registry surviving much beyond its centenary. In this brave new world, I am surprised that no one has advocated that a polygraph should replace professional medical evidence. That would tell us whether the client was lying or not and would eliminate the problem of non-disclosure.

Sadly, from my point of view, the Freedom to Underwrite is becoming a thing of the past. Indeed, with all these threats, life offices may withdraw from the protection market. That really could place a burden on the state.

APPENDIX 1.1

Report of the Select Committee on Science and Technology

The House of Commons appointed the Science and Technology Committee in 1992. The committee's third report, *Human Genetics: The Science and its Consequences*, was published on 6 July 1995. The issues relating to genetic tests and life insurance were of particular interest to the committee. Concerns about the industry were raised by a leading geneticist, Professor Peter Harper, the British Diabetic Association and the Genetic Interest Group. Dr Nicholas Barr from the London School of Economics looked at the issues independently and gave evidence. The report is of crucial importance to the future of the industry and so, with the kind permission of HMSO, I am reproducing most of the section on insurance. The committee chose to put some sentences in bold type, which is repeated here.

235. Many of our witnesses were very concerned that the availability of genetic information might have profound effects on the insurer as well as the insured. Knowledge of the results of a genetic test showing susceptibility to a serious illness gives an incentive to that person to take out a life insurance. To avoid adverse selection of risks, insurance companies now require the insured to give the results of any genetic test they may have had, but do not require that any further tests be made. An adverse result from a test may increase the premium required, or may make insurance unobtainable. This in turn gives an individual an incentive to avoid having a genetic test. Such avoidance may imperil the health and well being of the insured and of their families. In seeking a solution which resolves the problem, it is useful to consider who should bear which costs. At present the individual may bear the cost of

higher premiums or the non-availability of insurance, or incur a risk to health. If insurance companies did not seek or use available information on the results of genetic tests, individuals, knowing they were going to die early, could take out large insurances, and the costs of the higher premiums would fall on the general body of the insured. There is some benefit to the insured generally in that they would know that in the future they would not be discouraged from taking otherwise desirable genetic tests by the cost of new insurances. But there is a cost in higher premiums. The problem is to seek arrangements that balance the costs and benefits.

It is interesting to re-read this section, substituting the words 'medical test' for 'genetic test' in the appropriate places. No one would argue that a medical test for heart disease should be kept from an insurance company. Genetic tests are medical tests, and yet the thrust of the argument is that they are somehow different from other tests. Are they, and should someone who has had a genetic test as opposed to a medical test for some other reason be treated differently?

At present, proposal forms do not mention genetic tests. They do, however, require proposers to give details of any medical tests they have undergone. The wording, 'insurance companies now require the insured to give the results of any genetic test they may have had', indicates that the select committee accepts that it would be non-disclosure if a proposer failed to convey this information and it was not covered by an agreement to waive it.

> 236. This is not solely a United Kingdom fear; in the Netherlands, there has been a moratorium which bans the use by insurance companies of the results of information from genetic tests for applicants for life and private genetics – the disability insurance is up to Fl 200,000 (£81,300). This moratorium has recently been renewed and the Government has asked insurance companies to revise their policy of not covering those with a family history of muscular dystrophy or Huntington's disease. Discussions on the implications of genetics for health insurance have been held in the USA.

The effect of the ban in the Netherlands means that proposers are able to withhold relevant information from insurance companies – and the companies are obliged to meet claims as they arise. It is difficult to determine the overall cost of such concessions, as individuals with a genetic disorder could be advised to effect life policies. In the long run, the additional claims would be paid by the policyholders themselves through increases in premium rates both for new policies and, where possible, for the revision of existing ones. If the premiums increase, those at high risk from a genetic disorder may still apply for policies but those at low risk may decide not to, hence escalating the problems for offices.

Taking this a stage further, a salesman could legitimately visit hospices signing up many of the occupants. Notices might even be placed in doctors' waiting rooms. Even the industry's most vicious critics should realise that this is untenable. Also, some people may learn that they are at high risk from cancer and some may learn that they are at low risk. Those at high risk are far more likely to want insurance.

If genetic history is banned on proposals, adverse selection becomes a major issue. How can discrimination against life offices by those who know they are high-risk be controlled? If the average sum assured is £50,000, those at higher risk may request £250,000, with the remaining policyholders effectively paying for that risk.

A ruling would be necessary, and suppose it was 'Every UK citizen between the ages of eighteen and sixty is entitled to £50,000 insurance but only accidental cover is available during the first year of the policy.' Should offices band together so that the first £50,000 of everyone's insurance is at a particular rate? It would be expensive to develop a register to show exactly who had proposed for what, and so those at greater risk could insure themselves with a range of offices. What, too, is to be done about existing cover at the introduction of such a ruling?

One way to avoid a register would be to have the proposer sign a declaration to say that this was the only concession he was applying for. At the time of a death claim from a genetic disease, offices could be circulated by a central source and payment delayed for a week to see whether any other offices respond positively. Delaying the payment of death benefits and the potential cutback in the overall amount could have negative repercussions on the industry.

All concessions have their costs and, to quote a leading actuary, David Purchase, in *The Times*, 'If society wishes certain adverse consequences to be avoided, society itself should pay the bill.' Yes, true, but it is unlikely that the government would give the industry financial support if such a moratorium proved costly.

237. If a genetic test predicted the future with sufficient accuracy, genetic information could, in theory, undermine the whole concept of insurance; as Dr Nicholas Barr, of the London School of Economics, said, 'The insurance industry cannot cope with certainty.' In practice, this is unlikely to happen. At the moment, as the Association of British Insurers (ABI) pointed out, there are few genetic tests available, and those are for serious conditions. No test is entirely certain, but these tests show whether or not a particular condition will develop to a very high degree of probability. However, some of our witnesses expected more extensive genetic tests for a far wider range of disorders to be introduced in the next decade. In fact, since screening or testing is likely to be introduced to identify those with a genetic predisposition to certain diseases, rather than those who will certainly develop them, all it is likely to do is to give more information about an individual's risk. We must also remember that, however accurate genetic testing may be about disease, people are always at risk of accident. Nonetheless, Dr Barr told us: 'My experience as somebody who studies the economics of insurance is to say that if the effectiveness of genetic testing spreads as widely as we are told, then that will have very major implications for insurance very quickly.'

A textbook could be written on the first sentence alone. People are going to die not only of genetic disorders but also from accidents, infectious diseases and the consequences of their life style. Furthermore, the ages of death of those with defective genes cannot be predicted. In any event, the insurance industry is able to cope with certainty. If someone has a twenty-five-year mortgage, a policy can be effected to pay it off at the end of the term. Irrespective of social considerations, the industry should welcome genetic tests, as they could add more accuracy to the pricing of risks.

238. In their evidence to the Committee, the ABI said that '... insurers do not require applicants for insurance policies to undergo genetic tests and they have no intention of doing so in the foreseeable future. However, insurance companies

do expect their clients to reveal the results of any genetic tests they may have undergone, and failure to do so could invalidate the policy.'

Quite so. It would be informative to have counsel's confirmation on *uberrima fides* and that non-disclosure of a genetic test constituted non-disclosure.

> 239. It is clear that some insurers have more experience in dealing with particular disorders than others, and that the industry does consider the opinions of professional geneticists when drawing up its assessment of risks. Individual medical officers of insurance companies also seem to have responded positively when geneticists have contacted them on behalf of particular patients. However, witnesses were concerned that, even at present, insurers were not able to interpret the relatively simple genetic information available to them. While there were no comprehensive studies to the extent to which genetic information was misinterpreted to a person's disadvantage, several cases in which this clearly had occurred were drawn to our attention.

The committee says that several cases of incorrect underwriting have been drawn to its attention and I would like to know where they came from. If it is argued that life offices are not able to interpret 'relatively simple genetic information', is it not possible that some geneticists do not appreciate the long-term nature of life insurance, the guarantees of premiums and the particular policies we have to underwrite?

> 240. If insurers are unable to deal with the simple tests available today, how will they react to the more complex tests which may soon be introduced? The insurers, in the main, were sanguine . . .

Following on from the last paragraphs, if these tests become so complex, just who will be able to understand them? It is not only the chief medical officers of the insurance companies who need educating but also every family doctor. If, on the other hand, the tests are so complex that they would not be able to interpret them, what is the point of doing them at all? Why should the government fund tests that can be understood only by a handful of geneticists?

My guess is that the committee has been heeding too many geneticists. If they are promoting their own specialty, has the committee a balanced view of the medical profession?

241. Opponents claimed that individual insurers might overreact to the mention of a genetic test on a proposal form, particularly in the early stages of genetic testing when such tests were associated with research programmes and their results were unclear. If this were to be the case disclosure of genetic tests to insurers could mean, as the Genetic Interest Group said:

> the advantages and risks of knowing one's risk are balanced with the advantages and risks of not knowing. For example, people with hypercholesterolaemia suffer from early onset heart disease, resulting in permanent disability and early death. If they are not identified as having a genetic disorder they can get life insurance, or be employed despite the fact that their health prognosis is extremely poor. Yet if they are listed, and follow the appropriate diet and medical care, they should be able to live a normal life style. However, they will be severely penalised by many insurance companies and often by employers too.

Reading this, there is a possibility that a cholesterol test could be regarded as genetic. Rather than enter that debate, the industry needs to state, 'These are the tests we rely on at present – ECGs, x-rays, HIV, blood profiles, urinalysis. We do not regard any of them as genetic tests.'

242. Although the ABI said, 'there are a very great number of . . . considerations of a social and of a personal nature before you go into screening . . . Insurance must be way down the list,' we understand that discussion of insurance is included in much genetic counselling. We accept that the insurance industry has collectively tried to deal with genetics in a responsible way; nonetheless we are concerned there is a real danger that people could decide to decline genetic testing, even when such testing would be advantageous to them, because of the possible insurance implications. Not only will this act to the detriment of those

directly concerned, but such reluctance could also hinder the research which will be needed if genetic knowledge is fully to benefit society.

I would like to know what is said about insurance in genetic counselling. Is it balanced and accurate? Judging by the counsellors for AIDS I have heard at insurance conferences, there is a misunderstanding of life insurance, despite the ABI's explanatory leaflets. This time the ABI should produce leaflets and, in exchange for the concessions, ensure that they are used.

The argument is similar to HIV testing – someone may not present himself for testing because he may have to declare it on a proposal in the future. It would be good for the industry if people did think of insurance so often, but, despite the advent of direct line insurance, insurance is sold rather than bought. I don't believe this is a problem for the individuals themselves, although pressure groups maintain it is.

243. Although insurance companies do not require genetic tests at present, some witnesses suggested that if one firm attempted to 'cherry-pick' by offering low rates to those with good genetic profiles others would be forced to do so. This would raise a number of ethical difficulties. Glasgow University Law Unit suggested that:

> the insurance companies will in effect force individuals to undergo testing which they might otherwise have chosen not to do. Insurance companies do not at present possess the necessary follow-up counselling procedures and care to educate people as to the relevance of this information.

When the Nuffield Council in Bioethics investigated genetic screening in 1993 it called for a moratorium on the use of genetic information in insurance policies below a certain threshold, and many geneticists and patients' interest groups have supported its proposal. Professor Harper told us that the insurance industry had been urged to hold discussions with the professions in genetics and the Department of Health. In May we were told that discussions between the ABI and geneticists were now being arranged and a meeting with genetic interest groups had already been held. We welcome this and hope it will mark the beginning of continuing contact between the insurers and those concerned with genetics research and treatment.

At present, underwriters prefer a pooled approach, where a wide number of people are covered at standard premiums and only those who are clearly abnormal are charged special terms or refused insurance. Life offices may want to keep this stance or change their approach.

244. The insurance industry's objections to a moratorium on the use of genetic information are based on the fear of adverse selection. Although genetic knowledge will not change the risk pool in the population as a whole, it will give people access to indications of their health prospects. If they do not have to reveal the results of genetic tests to insurers (and, one assumes, consequently pay a higher premium if appropriate), then those with bad prospects are more likely to insure themselves than those with good. The risk pool among the insured may be changed for the worse and insurance premia may rise. A vicious circle could be created if the risk pool deteriorated still further because those with good health prospects became increasingly reluctant to take out (expensive) insurance. We were told that this had indeed happened in the recent past:

> the insurance industry did a bold thing in the early 1980s. In terms of mortgage protection policies a number of companies at that stage decided that if a person was taking out a mortgage they could offer the cover without health evidence; . . . the evidence is that the mortality rate of those lives is broadly fifty per cent higher . . . than the normal insured life . . .

I know that Dr Pokorski in the US has had difficulty in establishing that adverse selection exists. It is, after all, something that insurance companies go out of their way to avoid. Some good has come out of the mistaken assumptions surrounding the MIRAS (mortgage interest relief at source) campaign in the UK, where business was accepted with no underwriting whatsoever. The high mortality experience illustrates the folly of the industry's concession. It shows that adverse selection exists.

245. Adverse selection is a real problem. Dr Barr admitted:

> Any sensible individual knowing they have got an un-
> favourable genetic predisposition will insure, and will
> insure as much as they are allowed to, and it is a
> matter for public policy to decide to what level they
> should be, if you like, entitled to insure.

246. We discussed possible solutions to the problem of adverse selection with Professor Kenneth Arrow, the Nobel Laureate economist, of Stanford University, and Dr Barr. One suggestion put to the Committee was that

(i) Insurance companies should not ask for any information or genetic tests at the time the contract was made.
(ii) If the insured dies of a genetic disease on a list maintained by an appropriate authority as predictable by
a genetic test, then the sum paid by the insurance company need not exceed a ceiling specified at the time of
the contract.
(iii) Insurance companies would re-insure in an industry
pool against the risks of deaths from genetically identifiable causes on the list.

The effect of this would be to spread the cost of payments from the genetically determined diseases on the list over the whole population of the insured. They would in turn gain from the knowledge that, in a rapidly moving field, they would not be discouraged from taking otherwise desir-able genetic tests by the cost of new insurances. Such a scheme would need detailed study and design. **The evidence given to us by Professor Arrow and Dr Barr suggests that it would be possible to find ways to regulate the use of genetic information in insurance which would both protect the inter-ests of society in enabling as many people as possible to obtain insurance and protect the insurance companies them-selves.**

Assume that a family man and breadwinner effects a policy to cover his mortgage for £250,000. Three years later he dies. If the disease is not on the list, the full £250,000 will be paid and the mortgage will be redeemed. If the disease is on the list, the sum assured may be reduced to £50,000, even though he will have paid premiums based on the higher sum assured. The lender may be forced to reclaim the property and the family will have to move.

There is also the unpredictability of this approach. No one knows how they are going to die, and the family will be able to claim the full amount if someone has a fatal accident just before the genetic disease goes into its final stages. Who is to say that all the deaths will really be accidents?

If this approach becomes the norm, how accurately will deaths be recorded? At the present time, AIDS is underrecorded and suicides are often classed as accidents. What pressure will a doctor be under to record a different cause of death such as heart failure and to omit the genetic component?

The definition of what is a genetic disease is increasing all the time and the list may become increasingly long. It would be unreasonable for someone who effected a policy in the year 2000 and died in the year 2010 to have his cause of death matched against the 2010 list.

The solution of a reassurance pool hardly helps the insurers. The funding for such pools has to come from somewhere – admittedly, the cost would be spread across several companies, but the total loss to the industry would be the same. We might question the use of reassurance at all if the sum assured is being limited.

There is another flaw in the argument. What if we request a medical attendant's report at the outset and the GP tells us the result of a genetic test?

I do not like this approach and think it would be far better to assess the risk at the outset, charge the appropriate premium and stick with it.

247. We cannot see into the future; it may be that the ABI is correct, and that the use of genetic information in insurance is limited, and raises no new problems. However, the great majority of our witnesses, including those with expertise in genetics, think that such information could have major implications for the industry in a relatively short time. In our view the ABI has reacted to these predictions with undue complacency; it would, at least, be prudent to have contingency plans in place to ensure that changes were dealt with in an orderly manner.

248. Such plans may now be being made. When we met the ABI we were told that the industry hoped to make its own proposals for dealing with genetic tests in 1995. **The Committee recommends that the insurance industry be**

allowed one year in which to propose a solution acceptable to Parliament, and that if it fails to do so a solution should be sought, by legislation if necessary.

249. Our proposal is limited to genetic information. Professor McLean pointed out that allowing use of family histories gave insurers access to a considerable amount of genetic information, and that there needed to be wholesale consideration of the use of medical information in insurance. She believed that we should accept that premia would increase in the interests of equity. This may happen in the long term; however, in the short term, like Dr Barr, we stand by 'pure, grubby empiricism': the extra premia currently charged affect only a relatively small number of people; the implications of genetic testing may however be much wider.

Life offices have asked about family history for years, and it is particularly relevant to critical illness policies, where payment is made on the diagnosis of a heart attack or cancer. Some proposers will be charged extra premiums on the basis of a poor family history. Life offices would be reluctant to give up such questioning.

250. Our discussion has concentrated upon life insurance, since that is the most relevant in the UK. However, if the most optimistic forecasts are right, genetic knowledge could change the whole nature of health insurance by limiting the ability to spread risk. A recent study in the US suggested that 'information about past, present or future health status, including genetic information, should not be used to deny health care coverage or services to anyone', and indeed medical underwriting has already been forbidden in several states. Sir Walter Bodmer thought that any country that 'does not have some form of health service that spreads the insurance risk not as a function of an individual's constitution will not be able to benefit' from the advances of genetic medicine. Several witnesses commented, unprompted, that the existence of the National Health Service was likely to spare the United Kingdom some of the most acute of the problems genetic science is likely to engender. **We believe that one effect of genetic information may well be to limit the scope of medical insurance in the medium to long term. Certainly countries which wish to use genetic**

**information in healthcare to the full will need some social
health system such as the National Health Service.**

APPENDIX 1.2

The Disability Discrimination Act 1995

In November 1994 the government announced that it would be
introducing a Bill concerning discrimination on grounds of disability. The Bill aims to end unfair discrimination against disabled
people. In its White Paper the government said:

> The Government accepts that measures to end discrimina-
> tion must be comprehensive. The lives of disabled people
> cannot be compartmentalised into a series of separate activ-
> ities. Like everyone else, disabled people want to be allowed
> to live life to the full. Improved access to goods and services
> is of little use to someone who cannot get on the bus to go to
> the shops. Access to a good education is essential when
> competing in the job market. For these reasons, govern-
> ment action must affect all areas of life, including work,
> travel, study and leisure. In some areas, such as getting
> work or going shopping, legislation is needed to secure
> equal status for disabled people. In other areas, such as edu-
> cation, it is better to build on existing provision with prac-
> tical measures which improve access.

The then Minister for the Disabled, William Hague, said, 'The consultation document made clear the Government's intention to
exclude financial services from any right of equal access. But as a
result of responses received, I propose to include financial services
in the new statutory right. We shall be looking closely, in consultation with the insurance industry, at how legislation could be best
framed to prevent discrimination while recognising the legitimate
need for insurance companies to distinguish between any customers
on the basis of likely costs entailed in meeting their insurance
claims.'

Baroness Hollis of Heigham asked, 'May we hope that there is as
much toughness with regard to the provision of financial services as
to other aspects of the Bill?'

The Bill was published in January 1995. Over 200 amendments
were tabled and there was also a new private member's Bill, because

it was thought that the Bill did not go far enough. The Disability Discrimination Act 1995 made it 'unlawful to discriminate against disabled persons in connection with employment, the provision of goods, facilities and services or the disposal or management of premises; to make provision about the employment of disabled persons; and to establish a National Disability Council.'

> 1. (1) Subject to the provisions of Schedule 1, a person has a disability for the purposes of this Act if he has a physical or mental impairment which has a substantial and long-term adverse effect on his ability to carry out normal day-to-day activities.

In this context, the word 'substantial' has yet to be defined, while 'long-term' is defined as a minimum of a year. 'Normal day-to-day activities' covers such areas as mobility, manual dexterity, physical co-ordination, continence, the ability to lift, carry or otherwise move everyday objects, speech, hearing or eyesight, memory or ability to learn or understand and the perception of the risk of physical danger.

As I see it, there has to be a disability in place, that is, the disability has actually to manifest itself. This seems eminently sensible, but some will argue for those who are HIV positive and those with a poor genetic profile. The inclusion of either category would cause problems for insurers.

In any event, I would have thought it could be mentally harmful to treat currently healthy people as disabled. Lord Ashley would disagree: 'They are very vulnerable people; they are waiting for an illness. There is no excuse for the Government refusing them protection.'

Those with a poor genetic profile may decide against having a family, and this led to some brilliant logic from Earl Russell. 'The Minster argued that a genetic defect is not a disability. Parenthood is a normal activity. How far it is exactly to be described as a day-to-day activity, I am not exactly clear. However, I should have thought that within the meaning of the Act, arguing that case in court, I might have had a sporting chance.'

> 4. (1) It is unlawful for an employer to discriminate against a disabled person –

(a) in the arrangements which he makes for the purpose of determining to whom he should offer employment;

(b) in the terms on which he offers that person employment; or

(c) by refusing to offer, or deliberately not offering, him employment.

There are several sections on employment, and most of it is good common sense. It is clear that every job cannot be open to every person. It would be unthinkable to employ a blind fireman or a blind bus driver. Quite clearly, though, the number of disabled persons in employment will increase, and so there will be more disabled employees in group life assurance schemes provided by insurers.

19. (1) It is unlawful for a provider of services to discriminate against a disabled person –

(a) in refusing to provide, or deliberately not providing, to the disabled person any service which he provides, or is prepared to provide, to members of the public;

(b) in failing to comply with any duty imposed on him by Section 21 in circumstances in which the effect of that failure is to make it impossible or unreasonably difficult for the disabled person to make any use of any such service;

(c) in the standard of service which he provides to the disabled person or the manner in which he provides it to him; or

(d) in the terms on which he provides a service to the disabled person.

19. (3) The following are examples of services to which this section and Sections 20 and 21 apply –

(a) access to and use of any place which members of the public are permitted to enter;

(b) access to and use of means of communication;

(c) access to and use of information services;

(d) accommodation in a hotel, boarding house or other similar establishment;

(e) facilities by way of banking or insurance or for grants, loans, credit or finance;

(f) facilities for entertainment, recreation or refreshment;

(g) facilities provided by employment agencies or under Section 2 of the Employment and Training Act 1973;
(h) the services of any profession or trade, or any local or other public authority.

The Disability Discrimination (Services and Premises) Regulations 1996

The regulations are intended to give some of the practical detail necessary for the introduction of the Disability Discrimination Act. For the purposes of insurance, the main regulation is:

2. (1) Where, for a reason which relates to the disabled person's disability, a provider of services treats a disabled person less favourably than he treats or would treat others to whom that reason does not or would not apply, that treatment shall be taken to be justified for the purposes of Section 20 of the Act in the circumstances specified in paragraph (2).

2. (2) The circumstances referred to in paragraph (1) are that the less favourable treatment is:

(a) in connection with insurance business carried on by the provider of services;
(b) based on information (for example, actuarial or statistical data or a medical report) which is relevant to the assessment of the risk to be insured and is from a source on which it is reasonable to rely; and
(c) reasonable having regard to the information relied upon and other relevant factors.

In the White Paper the government had said, 'Insurance services will be subject to a special rule which recognises the need to distinguish between individuals on the basis of the risks against which they seek to insure. Insurers will be allowed to charge higher premiums only to the extent that the extra charge is based on actuarial data or other good reasons.' This has been expanded, but not to any great extent, in (b) above. I would think that the element of reasonableness will be open to interpretation. Offices will need to consider that mythical man on the Clapham omnibus.

On the whole, I do not see there being much difference in making day-to-day underwriting decisions, but I may be wrong. After all, any underwriter who makes a decision should be able to justify it. I expect that far more will have to be documented and that offices will need a rationale for the extra premiums they charge. It would then be hard to demonstrate that the decision-making processes were not reasonable.

The ABI has suggested a Statement of Practice:

- The need for insurers to be aware of the main forms of disability and whether they have any relevance in assessing the size and probability of an insurance claim.
- The need for insurers to be aware of the wide range of conditions which may amount to 'disability' as distinct from medical impairment.
- The need for insurers to be able still to reflect claims experience, mortality and morbidity or other relevant factors in their underwriting.
- The need for insurers to ask only for medical information which is demonstrably related to the additional risk associated with insuring the disabled person.
- The need for complaints from disabled people to be handled sensitively.
- The need for insurance companies to have a clear mechanism for the investigation of a complaint by a disabled person.

The ABI is bound to have extensive discussions with the Department of Social Security and the Department of Trade and Industry with the aim that insurers should be able to differentiate premiums on the basis of reliable data concerning relative risks.

Decisions will need to be made on objective information and, to that end, it would be mutually beneficial to have a database of information. It needs to be two-sided, as either side could otherwise just put forward the figures most favourable to their cause.

The ABI needs to contact disabled groups in order to encourage the emergence of any further information that may be of assistance to underwriters in assessing disabled lives. However, actuarial expertise will be needed to explain why a particular set of favourable statistics may not be appropriate, e.g. based on too small a sample.

The Institute of Actuaries has a role to play, particularly with its inter-office investigations into impaired lives. Although funded by the institute, the Continuous Mortality Investigation Bureau is an independent body reporting purely on mortality and morbidity statistics. If those statistics were unfavourable to the offices, they would still be published.

Although it may not be the Bill's intention, life offices may be reluctant to introduce new products. Innovation involves risk and assumes a step into the unknown. It may be hard to justify the 'good reason' for applying additional premiums, as appropriate data may not be available.

The government will provide free advice to complainants in disputes, so disabled people will be able to take insurers to court for damages. Damages for hurt feelings can be sought, although there will be an upper limit.

NOTES

1 The chapter represents my own views and should not be taken as representing the views of any office with which I have been associated. Nor does it represent the views of the Association of British Insurers (ABI), where I sat on the Life Assurance and Medical Affairs Committee. The Association of British Insurers is a trade association representing the interests of over 400 insurance companies. Over 95 per cent of the total life business in the UK is written with offices affiliated to the ABI. The ABI considers industry matters and makes recommendations to its members, after perhaps seeking guidance from chief executives. The ABI cannot enforce its recommendations, but they are usually accepted. I would expect that to be the case with the recommendations it makes on genetics and disability, whilst it has already happened with AIDS.

2 Here is a summary of the treatment of AIDS by insurers in other countries:

Australia. Following a government inquiry, insurers adopted a code of practice in 1988. The code ensures that no one will be declined for insurance on the basis of their sexual orientation alone, although its application has been questioned by AIDS pressure groups. The Commonwealth Disability Discrimination Act, introduced in 1993, makes it illegal to exclude someone from insurance or superannuation benefits where the act of discrimination is not based on actuarial evidence. It has been suggested that if the AIDS exclusion clauses imposed on superannuation benefits are tested in court, they may be deemed illegal.

Canada. According to the country's law on human rights, proposers for life assurance cannot be discriminated against either because they are gay or because they have been tested for HIV infection. A spokesman for the Canadian AIDS Society, an umbrella organisation of more than seventy community AIDS groups across Canada, has said, 'It's not a problem here. I don't know of any instance where insurance companies have turned people away or discriminated in any way against them because they have taken a test previously. Nor do I know of anyone being turned down or discriminated against on the basis of being in a high-risk group.'

Denmark. There are no questions about life style on the proposal form, and the Danish Medical Association has instructed doctors to 'only disclose information that is relevant, and this should not include a HIV negative test'. However, a proposer can obtain cheaper premiums by answering a questionnaire which asks about HIV tests taken in the previous ten years.

France. The Ministry of Health forbids questions about life style and it obliges offices to issue acceptance terms for policies covering mortgages to applicants who are HIV positive. The resulting business is pooled amongst direct offices and reassurers, but as the extra premium charged is large (around £60 per £1,000 sum assured per annum) there have not been many takers. The potential for victims proposing on their deathbeds must be worrying for the offices.

Italy. Following an agreement with the trade body, HIV testing takes place when the sum assured is over £135,000 or when it is merited by the medical evidence. Otherwise, there is an exclusion clause for death by AIDS during the first five years of a contract. If a proposer refuses to take a test, the exclusion clause is extended to seven years. Neither the authorities nor pressure groups have opposed this.

The Netherlands. Until 1993, proposers were asked, 'Have you ever undergone a blood test for sexually transmitted diseases such as syphilis or AIDS? If yes, why, when, for what and with what result?' Many objections to this question were raised, and after discussion in parliament, the Dutch Association of Life Insurers modified the questions to 'Have you got AIDS? Have HIV antibodies been found in your blood?' The government has accepted life offices requesting an HIV test automatically for larger sums assured (over £76,000).

Norway. No questions about life style are permitted but individuals can be asked if they have had a negative HIV test.

United States. The position is complex because legislation varies from state to state. Some states, for example, have insisted that HIV tests are taken before someone is given a driving licence or is getting married. It is against public policy to penalise people who have taken an HIV test because the United States wants to encourage testing. Life offices can request HIV tests but they cannot ask questions to determine whether a proposer is a member of a high-risk group. Some states have stricter legislation than others and, as a result, some offices have decided not to write business there.

3 Regulations or legislation governing the life assurance industry have come from non-governmental bodies such as the Nuffield Foundation's Council on Bioethics. It is in this climate that the Science and Technology Committee looked at the questions surrounding human genetics and life assurance. Initially, I was cautious about this. There was a danger of premature and ill-conceived regulations through the committee being persuaded by criticisms from the medics, the moralists and those who are 'genetically unfit' and consider they are being victimised. Baroness Warnock at the International Human Gene Mapping Conference said that legal safeguards must be established against compulsory genetic screening. She said, 'Insurance companies will demand a genetic printout as they now demand a medical examination, and the result will be

that people and their families may be compelled to discover things that they would have preferred not to know.' The word 'compelled' is wrong because no one is compelled to apply for life assurance.

4 The ABI published a new code of practice in December 1997.

Offices will not request genetic tests – at present, an unlikely occurrence anyway – and, for mortgage policies up to £100,000 sum assured, will not seek information about previous tests. This has to be accepted, of course, but it is illogical. Why should home buyers be given special consideration? Surely if there is going to be a concession, then it should apply to life cover for your dependants as well? A preference would be £70,000 for any life policies.

Ironically, the ABI recommendation, which has the approval of geneticists, could weaken confidentiality as an office needs to ensure that a genetically-impaired individual is not applying to a succession of offices for £100,000 cover with each.

Offices are still entitled to ask about family history, and individual underwriters may reach different conclusions when confronted with a family history of Huntington's Disease. The Genetics Advisor to the ABI may, for expediency, recommend a decision but this would remove the competitiveness between offices.

2

FREEDOM WITHIN LIMITS

Underwriting and ethics

Tom Sorell

Should private insurers be entirely free to decide what risks to take on, and free also to set high premiums for high risks? Other things being equal, the answer is 'Yes'. If all applications for insurance had to be approved no-questions-asked, or if high-risk applicants had to be treated the same as everyone else, payments to cover losses might quickly bankrupt firms, or keep them in business only by burdening the low-risk with unreasonably high charges. The survival of firms and the affordability of cover for the low or average risk could be threatened if the freedom to underwrite were taken away or significantly curtailed. But to say that the freedom to underwrite should normally be respected is not to say that it is absolute. It may be overridden or restricted, because it can conflict with goods that are more important than efficient insurance markets. This chapter is concerned with the limits of the freedom to underwrite, but it also has to do with the moral differences between different kinds of insurance, and with the very great moral risks associated with restricting access to medical insurance.

THE MORAL IMPORTANCE OF MEDICAL INSURANCE

Although it can sometimes be used to pay for treatment that is unnecessary or that has doubtful benefits, medical insurance also protects people against life-threatening, highly disabling, and extremely painful, conditions, and these are among the most uncontroversial examples of the bad things in life. It is widely agreed that medically serious conditions make particularly strong claims on resources, and

54

are a higher priority than other conditions, even when the other conditions are uncontroversially bad in turn. For example, it is hard to deny that poverty is bad; that unemployment is bad; that illiteracy is bad; yet the badness even of these things is eclipsed by the badness of catastrophic life-threatening disease, or the badness of intense, unrelieved pain. These are among the worst of the bad things, and to be without the resources to have something done about them when they arise is, by the same token, one of the worst things as well. Private insurance schemes provide the necessary resources; where there is no alternative to such schemes the misfortune of being uninsurable is very considerable – more considerable, arguably, than the misfortune of being charged high premiums when one is at low risk of making a medical insurance claim.

Other things that people take out insurance against, like the cancellation or curtailment of a holiday, are relatively minor misfortunes. Not to be protected against these risks, or not to be offered insurance against them at an affordable price, is far less serious than not having medical cover. And 'far less serious' means far less serious morally in particular. There is something faintly silly about the idea of a human right to holiday insurance, but the idea that everyone is entitled to be spared avoidable suffering or premature death seems to be moral common sense. To be entitled to get pain relief or medical treatment for cancer, one should not have to be wealthy or well brought up or morally admirable. Still less should treatment depend on being a good insurance risk. So it is unsurprising that there should be moral issues about the freedom to underwrite in medical insurance, even when there is no objection to a freedom to underwrite in general. Of course, many of these issues affect the services that medical insurance pays for even more directly than insurance itself. If freedom from pain and disease is as important a good as one gets, then it is wrong for the price of the treatment to be set higher than necessary by doctors, makers of pharmaceuticals and medical equipment, and so on. If insurance costs from these sources were lower, the costs of not underwriting would be lower, too. So the ethics of underwriting is not an ethics for insurers only.

It is not necessarily an ethics only for *private* insurers, either. If it is morally wrong for certain medical conditions to go untreated, then perhaps the availability of treatment cannot – morally cannot – be determined by market forces. Perhaps too much is left to chance when access to medical care is one product among others for consumers to choose, and when different firms compete with one another for a pool of low-risk policyholders. Market forces may encourage certain people who would be sold insurance if they applied for it to take the risk of having no cover, and market forces may similarly make other groups – the elderly poor, for example – uninsurable. One rationale for compulsory, state-run medical insurance schemes is that less is left to chance. The insurance pool includes everyone, regardless of the likelihood of someone's drawing on its funds. So the risks of the poor and ill can be relied upon to be borne partly by the wealthy and healthy. On the other hand, the pool is likely to be big enough and to have enough of a surplus of contributors over claimants to make the charges to everyone who pays affordable, and at the same time substantial enough to pay for morally urgent treatment, even treatment beyond the morally urgent. This effect more than counterbalances the compulsory nature of the scheme.

One of the most important questions for people who agree that medically serious conditions are morally compulsory to treat is whether a compulsory, state-run, universal medical insurance scheme is morally avoidable. In much of the West there is a consensus that it is *not* avoidable, that a medical insurance scheme ought to be at the heart of the welfare state, and that it should be funded out of taxation on individuals, or employers, or both. Private health insurance schemes typically coexist with state-provided ones, but where they do, the issues associated with underwriting are very different from the ones that arise in countries where medical insurance is mainly a private sector responsibility.

IS THERE A FREEDOM TO UNDERWRITE IN THE *ABSENCE* OF A STATE-RUN INSURANCE SCHEME?

The US stands out among the developed countries as a place where a compulsory state-run health insurance scheme has been resisted, and where there may be a pro-market consensus in the population at large, as opposed to the business community or the medical establishment. The insurance market in America is not just made up of for-profit firms; even not-for-profit firms underwrite some medical insurance policies, which makes cover unaffordable for some people if it is available at all. It is not true that such people are cut off from medical treatment altogether, but it is in short supply, of relatively low quality, and overused. Group insurance plans attached to one's employment afford some protection to the high-risk, for these plans do not all require extensive medical checks. But people outside these schemes who are judged high risks and have recourse only to the inadequate safety net for the American uninsured are obviously badly off.

Are people in America treated unjustly if they are refused insurance because they are high risks? This is a bigger question than it may seem, because one of the things at issue may be the right of Americans to reject what they call 'socialised medicine' and to affirm the free enterprise system or capitalism as an integral part of American democracy. If underwriting is necessary for the free enterprise system to extend to a market in insurance, and if the free enterprise system is widely endorsed, then perhaps the costs to the ill or poor of underwriting are tolerable, because, in the view of Americans, the free enterprise system has more benefits than costs. On the other hand, if delays in pain relief and the treatment of serious disease are not justified even by the existence of a majority in favour of free enterprise or private insurance markets; if there is always a right to pain relief and the treatment of disease where the means of treatment are not absent; then perhaps injustice is what there is.

Medical insurance losses due to the patient's negligence

No doubt the injustice is mitigated where the responsibility for the pain or disease is overwhelmingly the patient's, and where the pain and disease were readily foreseeable and preventable. Someone who ignores medical advice for years and smokes himself into lung disease; someone who takes no notice of medical instructions to diet, and who becomes obese and contracts diabetes, is responsible for becoming a high-risk insurance applicant. Such a person is guilty of injustice in the doctor/patient relationship, since it is for the patient as well as the doctor to promote and protect the patient's health. Such a person is also guilty of injustice in the setting of public health insurance, because one ought to be in solidarity with fellow members of the insurance pool, and that means not becoming a burden on the pool through negligence.[1] The conclusion is not that the lung disease or diabetes of the negligent patient does not call for treatment, but that there is not necessarily any injustice in that treatment not being readily forthcoming or in the payment not necessarily being forthcoming automatically. On the contrary, the injustice may be in the actions leading to the patient's contracting the disorder. In general, the greater the patient's responsibility in raising the risk of an insured loss, the greater the justification on the insurer's part for refusing to insure, or for contesting a claim under a policy. Having insurance against a loss is not a reason for making the loss more likely, nor is it an excuse for negligence. The insured is expected, and *reasonably* expected, to want to avoid the loss more than he wants to suffer it and get compensation. That means not taking unreasonable risks. Smoking too much and eating too much, now that so much is known about the effects, deserve to be regarded as high-risk activities like skydiving and mountain climbing. This is not to say that mountain climbers and skydivers who are injured should not be treated, only that there is no injustice in their being expected to bear some of the cost of the unnecessary addition they make to the burden on medical services. In the same way, it is not unjust that smokers should pay high taxes on cigarettes, or that obese people who want private health insurance should pay more for it than those who watch their weight.

Medical losses beyond one's control: genetics and underwriting

If it is wrong and not just unfortunate for people knowingly to impair their health; if the responsibility for increasing the risks of insured loss tells in favour of insurers' taking into account those increased risks, both at the stage at which a policy is issued and at the stage at which a claim is made under a policy, what are we to say where someone is at high risk of developing a medically serious condition and the source of the risk is *not* what a person does but his genetic inheritance? Is there less reason to hold the increased risk against the applicant for insurance, because there may be nothing he could have done to avoid it? The fact that insurers have long taken account of family history in fixing premiums for medical insurance shows that inheritance *has* been considered in under-writing. Not only that, but questions about family medical history have rarely been regarded as intrusive or inappropriate when put on proposal forms. Has it been fair to take into account factors affecting risk that are beyond people's control? Where it does not put medical cover entirely out of reach, or affect the price very much, it is hard to see any objection to it. After all, in other forms of insurance, unavoidable risk uncontroversially weighs in setting premiums. If you are born and brought up in a place that is prone to storms, and so need storm insurance, then, though neither the storms nor the greater incidence where you live, nor even your living there, is due to you, it is not unreasonable for you to be charged more than someone who lives in a place where storms are virtually unknown.

The really troubling case for underwriting and genetic inheritance is where having a certain genetic inheritance would guarantee you a possibly huge financial loss and where an insurer's knowing or having reason to believe as much would leave you uninsurable, with no resources at all to meet the loss. But, once again, the argument against underwriting in this case is not from your lack of responsibility for the insured loss, but from the nature of the medical condition that created the loss. That someone is going to suffer a painful, severely debilitating disease is a reason for him to be helped – *however* the disease was contracted. Responsibility for the disease makes the patient blameable for getting into the state where he needs the help, but does not alter the fact that help is what he needs. And for the disease to be genetic is for the patient blamelessly to need the help; it is not for the patient to need the help more than the one who is responsible for his condition. The severity of the need is the thing that makes the help compulsory, not the blamelessness of the need. If the condition is bad enough, the necessity of relieving it is not in doubt. But it does not follow from the fact that there is an obligation for *someone* to do something about the bad condition that it is a private insurer's responsibility to do that thing, or to waive risk assessment where the risk is due to factors beyond the applicant's control. It may be that what the argument shows is that there has to be a *public* insurer of last resort, or comprehensive and compulsory public insurance

Not that genetic conditions are bound to be uninsurable privately. Not that the private insurer has to ask for the fullest genetic information wherever there is a risk through genetic disease of an insured loss. As Spencer Leigh points out in Chapter 1, it is possible even for private insurers who exercise to the full the freedom to underwrite to relax risk assessment where an affordable upper limit is placed on insurers' liability.[2] As for tests, even where the science of genetics has made very accurate ones possible, insurers have sometimes been reluctant to require them. There is a potential marketing disadvantage in requiring tests, and the costs of test procedures themselves are a deterrent, since they have to be borne whether or not an insurance applicant ever ends up taking a policy.[3] Some of the diseases for which tests exist are extremely rare: an expensive test for a rare disease is unlikely to be a cost-effective means of minimising future claims. Again, a moderately cheap test for indications of more common sources of insured losses – cigarette smoking or alcohol consumption – may be expensive to conduct often. And even cost-effective tests are likely to discourage potential customers who would rather not know whether they have a serious genetic disease or a chance of developing its symptoms, or who dislike medicals. Insurers who insist on tests are likely to face competition from other companies who see the market opportunity of offering cover with relatively few questions asked. In life insurance markets as they are already known in the West, certain preferred risks – non-smokers in their thirties – are sometimes offered life policies with cover over $200,000 on the basis of a telephone conversation – with no medical examination at all. Such practices underline the fact that, in North America and the UK at any rate, insurance companies tend to want to write new business more than they want to avoid risk. As the Association of British Insurers likes to point out, 95 per cent of proposers of life insurance in the UK are offered policies on standard terms, and only 1 per cent of applications are refused.

Genetic diseases, then, do not necessarily raise greater difficulties for underwriting than other diseases, and when genetic diseases do raise big problems, it is typically because the diseases are serious, not because they are genetic. With only a few qualifications, it is possible to say that questions about the fairness of genetic underwriting do not add much to questions about the fairness of medical underwriting in general. But it is now time for the qualifications. The use of genetic information by insurers does make some difference. For one thing, genetic tests can establish with near certainty that certain conditions will be contracted, whereas family history may have left the question more open. For another, the implications of a genetic test spread beyond the person it is about: to other family members, whose insurance prospects may be harmed without their knowing, and without their being able to do anything about it. Again, and as with genetic research that has already taken place, there are strong temptations to link genetic profiles pretty speculatively with intelligence, adult criminal activity, life expectancy, athletic performance and many other things, but especially things that are financially profitable or costly – either for the individual or for society. Insurers, employers and others will have to decide how far it is prudent, profitable or right to accept or decline insurance proposals, set premium levels, hire and so on, on this basis, and some people who are disadvantaged by these speculations will also be wronged by insurance companies and other institutions.

No doubt other kinds of unfairness have already resulted from institutions giving credence to speculative psychological and sociological theories, so that genetic theories are just one more in a long line. It is arguable, however, that in the case of genetics the temptation to credit speculation will be stronger. Not only is the Human Genome Project making more people than ever aware of advances in molecular genetics; the growing awareness is an incentive to make further advances and quicken the already speeding maturity of genetics as a science. There is more than a small danger that the enormous, and still growing, authority of genetics will rub off on spurious genetic speculation, especially when the speculation feeds a commercial interest. It is no answer to say that in the long run the unfounded speculation will be weeded out. In the long run a lot of people can be denied the jobs they need and the insurance they need and may have run out of time to get compensation for unnecessarily lost opportunities. So it is necessary for everyone, the insurance industry included, to see to it that the burden of proof is sufficiently discharged.

HIV disease

An area where insurance companies may already have allowed unfair speculation to enter into underwriting decisions is the life and health insurance market for young single males since the identification of HIV deaths among homosexuals. Here the spectre of large numbers of huge pay-outs for protracted hospital care and expensive drugs, as well as premature deaths, has led insurers to ask for information that is widely thought to be unduly intrusive. Where the information has been given and insurance applications have been accepted, premiums have sometimes been heavily loaded – unduly heavily loaded, in the opinion of some insiders in the insurance industry, if only risk were being taken into account.

One question about underwriting in the HIV case is whether the right to privacy trumps the insurer's right to take on a risk only if relevant information is not withheld. The HIV case is delicate, because some of the information that is relevant – does a homosexual insurance applicant practise safe sex? – is about as personal as information gets, and well within the area that a right to privacy is supposed to protect. Questions about one's sex life seem much more intrusive than other personal questions that arguably violate a right to privacy but which are relevant to a firm's offering a commercial service. For example, if I have guaranteed my children's credit card debts, and then decide to apply for a big loan for myself, it is relevant for a commercial lender to ask me about my children's spending habits as well as mine, though they are not parties to the lending application; on the other hand, it is information about them, and theirs rather than mine to give out. A right to privacy certainly seems to be engaged by the lender's being very thorough in researching the risk of lending to me, even if the lending firm is not being nosy and is bored stiff by my children's financial situation. The thoroughness may even be obligatory: after all, the lender has legal and moral duties not to squander money on people who can't or won't repay, and so if he asks no questions he is in the wrong as well. Perhaps information about my children's spending can reasonably be *asked* for, even if I decide that I won't answer on the grounds that the question is intrusive. But some questions are so personal that even their being asked seems wrong. Suppose I apply for the loan at a time when I am about to get divorced. Divorce certainly has financial consequences. I may become unable to service debts I have barely managed to control before having to pay alimony or child support as well. If that is true, so that it is relevant to the lender's decision, hasn't the lender a right to know? The answer is 'No'. At most he has a right to ask. And in some cases even that right may not exist. After all, having children has financial consequences, but no one thinks that a lender may ask about a person's fertility and use of contraceptive techniques in order to calculate whether the expenses of having a baby will drive a couple into bankruptcy. On the other hand, there is nothing wrong with the lender's weighting applications from young low-paid people in couples for the possible financial consequences of having children, based on statistics for indebtedness for people of similar ages with similar jobs.

In the case of life or medical insurance where there is a risk of HIV disease, certain questions may also not be morally askable, relevant though they may be to predictions about claims under the policy. Thus there may be reasonable objections to a lifestyle questionnaire that tries to elicit information about the sexual habits of homosexual applicants. But if as a result of not having the questionnaire insurance companies load premiums, is that a reasonable or an unreasonable cost of not infringing privacy? Much depends, again, on whether after the loadings the insurance becomes unaffordable, and whether private insurance is the only protection against illness or premature death. If, as we have been assuming throughout this section, there is no reasonable public safety net to land on if private insurance is refused, unaffordability may be as intolerable as outright refusal. On the other hand, there seems to be no reason why there should not be voluntary trade-offs of privacy – say in the form of frank and full answers to lifestyle questionnaires – in return for very high potential life and health pay-outs, say over $500,000. In the same way, there could be relaxed underwriting, as in the genetics case, for policies under an affordable pay-out ceiling. That would meet Spencer Leigh's objections to insurance pay-outs in the millions in US jurisdictions that outlaw lifestyle questionnaires.[4]

Even this way of trying to strike a compromise between respect for the privacy of insurance applicants and reasonable commercial precautions against bad risks leaves the borderline between the intrusive and the reasonable question difficult to fix. The question of whether one has had an HIV test should not necessarily be unaskable: but positive answers to it cannot be taken as evidence of increased risk of HIV disease. If, out of fear of how the answers to the question will be unreasonably interpreted, large numbers of people either refuse to take the test or lie about having had it or about the results, no purpose is served by including it on a questionnaire. But, that said, there is no reason why people who have taken the test and know that they are HIV negative should not be able to use those facts to establish their status as a preferred risk under insurance schemes that are not blinded by prejudice about, for example, homosexual life styles. There is a niche, and perhaps a big one, for insurers that homosexuals can trust, just as there is a niche for property developers and night-club owners who are sympathetic to the justified fears of violence, financial manipulation and other sorts of offences to which homosexuals are exposed.

If it is not necessarily morally wrong to ask about the results of HIV tests, is it morally wrong to require such tests as a condition of insurance, employment or other things? Not if HIV testing occurs without a system of counselling for those whose results are positive; and not if positive results throw people back on an inadequate safety net. Finding out that one is HIV positive, at least until extremely recently, meant finding out that one would be destined sooner or later, and maybe quickly, to a debilitating and painful death, a death made worse by the ostracism reserved for a highly infectious disease carried by people sometimes thought to be sexually depraved. Going through a process in which one is prepared to find out that one has this dreaded condition is probably itself something of an ordeal, even if it is carried out by sympathetic counsellors. People should not lightly be required to undergo that process, however vital the test may be to underwriting, and however unlikely it is on balance that anyone who takes the test will suffer from the disease. And this is to say nothing of the money costs of a reliable and properly resourced testing and counselling system.

New developments, and ancillary issues in HIV insurance

HIV and AIDS used to be regarded as untreatable, highly disabling diseases, rendering their sufferers very weak, highly dependent and incapable of normal life and work. Now that drugs are available to counter the disease in its earliest stages and to control it once it is established, the idea of a privately insurable HIV disease sufferer is no longer inconceivable. On the contrary, on 15 April 1997 a small insurance company in the American state of Illinois, Guarantee Trust Life Insurance, started to offer policies to HIV positive patients. The maximum pay-out for policies was $250,000, for which the monthly premium for a non-smoking 'fairly healthy' thirty-year-old was $1,500. For coverage of $50,000 a thirty-year-old non-smoking policyholder had to pay $300 per month, about six times the monthly cost to someone without HIV disease.

Guarantee Trust Life was not prepared to treat all HIV positive applicants in the same way. Those who contracted the disease through needle stick injury or through sex were an acceptable risk, but intravenous drug users were not. The Guarantee Trust scheme thus recognises what is often missed in popular discussions of AIDS and insurance, that groups forming the potential market for HIV insurance are diverse. A market that insurers have tried to develop, sometimes aggressively in the UK, is that made up of health care workers. This market presents some distinct moral risks, because some people at low risk of contracting AIDS may be frightened into buying such insurance, and many health care workers, at least in the UK, are very low paid, and cannot afford it. Like the Guarantee Trust scheme, many of the schemes aimed at health workers exclude cover for certain sources of AIDS. Intravenous drug use may be an excluded source under one scheme; sex may be an excluded source under another. Where the pay-outs under policies are large, or in the event of many claims being made under policies with relatively low maximum pay-outs, there may be some incentive within the system to contest claims on the pretext that the source of the disease was on the excluded list, and to load premiums even more substantially to waive exclusions from some sources of HIV disease. If suffering HIV disease continues to carry the stigma it carries with it at the moment, the unpleasantness of contested insurance claims in general may be compounded in the case of these policies.

People with AIDS or who are diagnosed HIV positive may have a greater need of money at the end of their life than beneficiaries under their life policies would have after they die. In cases like these it is sometimes possible, and in any case morally desirable, for HIV positive policyholders with short life expectancy (two years or less) to be able to sell their policies for a high proportion of their full value. In the UK one such scheme[5] has proved practicable. Indeed, it has been a model of good practice. The organisation concerned advises applicants to get independent financial advice, operates a cooling-off period during which sellers of life policies can return the sum they have been paid and get their policies back, and makes no judgements about how people want to use their money. Finally, it adds no penalties if they survive beyond the two-year period of life expectancy.

Selective disclosure and the management of risk

In considering the ethics of insurance it is natural to put the individual insurance applicant in the role of David opposite the Goliath of an insurance company. Especially if the insurer has a long record of high profits, why should it not be deprived of some information about applicants that would enable it to minimise its already successfully controlled risks still further? Why should it not be deprived of this information, including the results of genetic tests or HIV tests, if gathering it and making it available are intrusive anyway, if it is information whose effects are likely to add to the disadvantage of people who are ill, and if the losses from risks can be borne without driving the company out of profit?

The idea that insurance losses fall only on institutions, and that the institutions are probably already too rich, is widespread. People who would not dream of keeping the extra change that the neighbourhood shopkeeper gives them through oversight are often quite prepared to inflate their losses on insurance claims, because the company is thought to be impersonal, faceless and large, with a size and shape so different from that of the local shopkeeper that it cannot feel personal financial pain. Businesses, even big businesses, are not like that, and some insurance companies are very far from being like it, having kept up some of the traditions of the co-operative association, or specialising in risks in the not-for-profit or public sector. In mutual insurance companies, where premium income is the sole or main source of claims, any pressure that increases claims puts upward pressure on premium levels and gives added reason for pervasive and accurate risk assessment based on the burdens of individual policyholders. People like the local shopkeeper feel the insurance company's pain. In insurance companies funded out of the proceeds of premiums and investment or other income, the effects of big losses arising from concealed risk or fraud are also higher premiums for policyholders and lower returns to shareholders. The shareholders need not be tycoons or large profit-making institutions. They can be local shopkeepers, or, differently, the pension funds of people who have no shares and small savings.

It is sometimes true that insurance fraud is perpetrated against rich companies, even ones that overcharge for policies or make questionable savings by contesting defensible insurance claims. This does not turn fraud into permissible activity, any more than robbery is made right by the fact that some people who are robbed came by their money or goods dishonestly or ruthlessly. Perhaps in the same way selective disclosure to insurers is bad, for reasons similar to those that might be brought up against lying. Politicians who self-servingly defend a policy of being economical with the truth are an object of contempt. Why should selective disclosure by private individuals not put *them* in the wrong as well? There is a difference, admittedly, between refusing to disclose information that would raise one's insurance premium and lying one's head off about one's insurance losses. For one thing, the refusal may have nothing to do with the higher insurance premiums: it may be based on the reasonable belief that the information requested is too personal to be asked for. Still, there is a background fact that connects non-disclosure and lying, and which insurers make much of, namely the huge asymmetry between what the insured knows about his losses and potential losses and what the insurer knows or can find out cost-effectively, if at all. When it comes to knowledge about losses or potential losses under a particular policy, the insurer is David and the insured is Goliath.

May one asymmetry – the knowledge asymmetry – counterbalance the other asymmetry – in financial strength and sophistication – between insurer and insured? If the asymmetries do cancel one another out, and parties to insurance contracts accept the asymmetries as a fact of life, there is a presumption in favour of not disturbing the balance too much. The more that insurance companies try to make up for the knowledge deficit by intrusive questioning, or by raising premiums across the board, the more the balance is disturbed, just as the balance is disturbed the more that policyholders try to stay ahead of the cost of premiums through fraudulent claims or non-disclosure in insurance applications. If considerations about maintaining this balance were decisive in insurance ethics, there would be a strong presumption in favour of not allowing health and life insurers suddenly to increase their powers of discovery through genetic tests, and a strong presumption in favour of life and health policyholders not weakening the financial position of companies through fraudulent claims or misleading insurance applications. But, of course, as things are, there are other destabilising forces in the insurance market – notably the increasing costs of treatment resulting from innovation, and the increasing costs of treatment resulting from increased demand.

These forces give an incentive to companies, especially in the health insurance market, to raise premiums and screen out risks even if all policyholders are honest and informative when asked to be. The same forces give policyholders an incentive to evade the screening and to be selective in their disclosure of information relevant to risk. Those who are excluded by screening techniques and who are poor are likely to add to the already big burden on public health services. Such people are forced to cope with the problems of belonging to a health care underclass in addition to having to cope with membership of an economic underclass. Against this background it is not just economically but morally important to control health costs. There is some evidence, however, that when the controls take the form of incentives to doctors to act as insurers' gatekeepers in the health care market, other moral risks are run. Doctors who send their patients for expensive tests or to hospital may be penalised by Health Management Organisations, and there is sometimes pressure to keep treatment times as short as possible. It may be that in the rich, industrialised countries the most cost-effective as well as least morally objectionable way of dealing with health insurance is by non-market means – by a universal, compulsory health insurance system, with contributions geared to ability to pay. Under these arrangements the insurance pool is large enough to make it likely that the rich and healthy will be able to pay for the ill and poor, and the risk of mortality or ill health is not made the ground of a lighter or heavier financial burden. Under these arrangements the side costs of a genetic disorder or predisposition are minimised without concealment, and the enforced sharing of risk is in a cause everyone can agree is good. As the cases of the UK and Canada show,[6] a public health insurance regime can not only deliver high-quality modern treatment, it can coexist with a profitable life insurance market and, for the wealthy, a small but profitable private insurance market as well.

UNDERWRITING IN THE PRESENCE OF A PUBLIC INSURANCE SYSTEM

If the moral importance of refusals of commercial insurance increases with the relative size of the private sector in insurance and medical care, what are we to say about the refusal of insurance, or setting commercial premiums high, in countries with big public sector health regimes? Is it morally important to have access to the commercial insurance market even in countries like these? As regards the UK the answer is 'Yes', because commercial life insurance or income protection insurance is often required to secure a loan to buy housing, to provide income during a period of illness if one is self-employed, or to provide for loss of income when an income earner or *the* income earner in a household dies. Private *medical* insurance is another matter. It makes a difference mainly in relation to speed of treatment for elective procedures, and to the provision of extras, such as private rooms, and certain sorts of meals, in hospitals. To be refused private health insurance when there is good public provision may be inconvenient and painful, given the waiting times for non-urgent conditions, but it is not morally intolerable, as the refusal of all health insurance is. So the freedom to underwrite is wider as well.

When it comes to life insurance, whether taken as desirable in itself or as a means to home ownership or something else, the moral issues surrounding underwriting conform to a pattern that has already emerged. How free insurers are to underwrite depends mainly on how morally bad it is for people to be denied the relevant form of insurance. It is disputable whether not to be a home owner is a big misfortune if one can rent property, even luxurious property, instead. And although it is much clearer that it is bad for the main earner in a family to die when he or she has dependants, the moral intolerability of not having life insurance to cover that loss depends again on the kind of safety net that exists for the uninsured. In a society in which there are generous state-provided widows' and widowers' pensions, and a system of payments for child support, the lack of commercial life insurance is perhaps not tragic. Similarly in the case of countries where there are strong customs of families or local communities helping the widowed and orphaned. Similarly again where the money that might have gone into paying for an insurance policy can be grown through investment to pay for death. Where none of these things is available, there is a moral argument for erecting or improving the public safety net or limiting the scope for private underwriting. But where either a safety net exists or means of saving are available that meet the demands of premature death, strict underwriting by private insurers may not matter so much.

Does public provision have moral costs?

I have written throughout as if, whatever the financial costs of the public safety net, it had no moral costs, and as if, at least in the case of medical insurance, the moral challenges could effectively be met only through a public health insurance scheme. It is perhaps time to draw back and ask whether moral costs are in fact absent in the provision of the safety net itself. If the costs are there, and if they are significant, they may constitute an argument against the freedom to underwrite in addition to the misfortune to the uninsurable of having no protection against serious illness or premature death.

It is sometimes thought that extensive safety nets are too inviting, and that more people than necessary make use of them. Thus the phrase 'dependency culture' has crept into the rhetoric of those who think that people in the UK should be more self-reliant – more dependent in particular on private provision for illness, death and old age. Again, and in the same vein, there are those who think that the taxation required to pay for the safety net reduces the entrepreneurial activity, and in some sense the freedom, of those who pay the taxes. Perhaps it also reduces their welfare, since if they had more to spend they could cater better for their personal preferences. Finally, there is a special version of the attack on dependence that suggests that there is a wilfully opportunistic minority who deliberately behave as free-riders, taking advantage of expensive benefits that they do not really need and which they are too lazy to go out and work for and pay for through taxation or privately. According to this line of thought, the free-riders are guilty of a sort of injustice which only the provision of less of a safety net – less of an opportunity for parasitism – will cure.

Though I am unsympathetic to such views, this much at least can be conceded to them: people who do not need to use the safety net should not use it. That leaves open the question of how many people (in the UK or elsewhere) use it needlessly. Unless the number is big and there are uncontroversial criteria of unnecessary use, the claim that there is a dependency culture, and the claim that the safety net encourages it, will remain tendentious. Clearly there are fraudulent and manipulative users of public health and welfare services, and the moral argument for prosecuting and eliminating free-riding of their kind is widely accepted and reflected in law in many welfare states, including the UK. What is far from clear is that shrinking the welfare state is a justified response to such free-riding over and above measures against fraud. Again, the moral condemnation of manipulation at the user end of the public welfare schemes has to be taken together with fraud at the contribution end, that is, tax fraud. It also has to be taken together with unequal access to tax loopholes, as well as the morality of exploiting such loopholes at all.

All that said, there *are* moral risks, and, when they are realised, moral costs, associated with the existence of a safety net, especially a safety net in the form of no-questions-asked comprehensive public health insurance. These moral costs do not, however, argue for widening the private insurance market or for restrictions on the scope for underwriting. The moral risks arise from greed on the part of providers of goods and services paid for by public insurance, negligence or selfishness on the part of users of those services, and overambitiousness in the spread of care. Let us consider these briefly in turn.

The National Insurance health insurance pool does not just buoy up those who are ill and otherwise in need of health care; it also pays for products that make already hugely profitable companies more profitable, and already wealthy consultants and managers even wealthier. It adds to the profits of the very large pharmaceutical multinationals, and of manufacturers of medical equipment and supplies. The less the non-needy take from the pool the more the needy can benefit from it. If this means that ceilings have to be put on managers' and consultants' salaries, or even those of GPs; if price controls have to be applied to health products; then that may be justified by the consequences for patients. But – and now we come to the second and third sources of moral risk – patients must do their part, and the service should not conspire in raising expectations about what services or levels of service are due to the public as a matter of right. Patients who abuse, or are violent with, medical staff, who ignore medical advice and yet develop the conditions they are warned about, who declare medical emergencies where none exists, are not meeting the requirements of justice that flow from belonging to a public insurance scheme, and are morally less urgent to treat than patients with identical conditions who do not abuse the system. At the violent end they should be treated only while under arrest and facing criminal charges. It is not as if the rationale of a public health care system has to extend to a rationale for abuses of the system by the medically needy. Unless 'abuse' is the wrong word because the behaviour it describes requires psychiatric treatment itself, there is no reason why people responsible for abuse should be ahead of non-abusers with the same medical problems in a queue for services.

Finally, the services should be free and widely available in proportion to the intolerability of the conditions they relieve. A public insurance system that paid for nothing that could be construed as elective would not necessarily be morally worse than one that gave a little, extremely expensive, elective treatment to the lucky few and in doing so took resources away from non-elective treatment. In the UK a wide array of elective treatments are available on the NHS, and some of them are expensive, not necessarily effective, and are not treatments for illness. Fertility treatment falls into this category. Although the unhappiness involved in not being able to conceive is considerable, infertility may not be urgent to treat when compared with cancer or correctable loss of eyesight or loss of mobility. Other treatments may be comparable in non-urgency. Even when they are available in a state-funded hospital system funded by contributions to a national health insurance scheme, it is not clear that they should cost the patients who want them nothing extra. On the contrary, the reasonableness of charging extra is directly proportional to the non-urgency of the treatment. Breast enlargements that are carried out merely to satisfy the wish of a woman or her partner are very high on the list of treatments for which patients should bear all or most of the cost. Perhaps there is some justification for a partial subsidy in the fact that, if certain elective treatments were left to pay for themselves, the skills needed for the relevant procedures might die out or be taught and never used. But there are limits to reasonable burdens on the resources of a national medical insurance scheme that eschews underwriting partly on the basis of the obligatoriness of treating the most painful and life-threatening conditions. When money from the pool is spent, the most painful and life-threatening conditions must always be given priority. It is true that an insurance system that covered a wider range of elective treatments free would be better when judged by *consumer* standards. But we confuse consumerism with morality at our peril.[7]

NOTES

1 See my 'Consumerism, ethics and the NHS reforms', *Journal of Medical Ethics* 23 (April 1997), 71–6.
2 Is there a way of striking a compromise between the supporters of full underwriting and the supporters of no underwriting, without ordinary premium payers being kept in the dark about the subsidies they are paying to the higher risk? One possibility I think would be worth market testing is the idea of an ethical insurance fund on the rough model of an ethical investment fund. In an ethical investment fund investors settle for lower returns on investments in companies that make money in relatively unobjectionable ways. In an ethical insurance fund, people would be charged higher than average premiums on the understanding that the difference between their premium and an ordinary premium would be used to lower the premiums of someone with a high-risk condition, or raise the number, or pay-out, of non-underwritten policies offered by the company. Another model for an ethical insurance fund would involve those with preferred lives (non-smokers, for instance, or those who have done well on genetic tests) entering an insurance pool at standard rather than discounted premiums, again with the idea of promoting non-underwritten policies or subsidising the premiums of the high-risk. Again on the model of ethical investments, insurance companies could track premiums with some contribution of their own to the reduction of margins, in order to convince potential policyholders of their good faith. I do not say that these products could be marketed to just anyone, but it would be interesting to see whether they attracted individual ethical investors or companies willing to insure even at standard rates with companies that tried to market convincing ethical insurance policies.
3 There is the further problem, at least in the UK, that few if any geneticists would be willing to carry out the tests for insurers. This was pointed out to me in correspondence by Spencer Leigh.
4 See Chapter 1 in this volume.
5 Run by Life Benefit Resources.
6 See Ted Marmor, *Understanding Healthcare Reform* (New Haven, Conn.: Yale University Press, 1994).
7 See note 1.

3

GENETICS AND ETHICS
The scientific background

Medical Research Council of the United Kingdom

GENETIC RESEARCH AND THE HUMAN GENOME PROJECT

1. What genetic research is carried out in the UK? How is it organised?

There is a strong tradition in the UK in human genetics, gene linkage and genetic technology. Indeed many of the basic technologies presently being used world wide for genome analysis were initially devised in the UK. Research on human genetic diseases is undertaken in many higher education institutions through funding from a variety of sponsors, as well as in directly supported establishments funded by the research councils and by certain of the charities. There is also increasing interest in genetics from the commercial sector.

Research in molecular and biochemical genetics has led to the development of novel recombinant DNA technologies which are providing new approaches to many unsolved problems, such as the organisation of genetic information, the regulation of embryonic development, differentiation, antibody production and vaccine development, as well as the molecular structure of proteins. Recombinant DNA techniques also permitted the production of proteins in cultured bacteria and cells, the isolation, analysis and manipulation of individual genes, detection of genetic defects leading to heritable conditions and ways of detecting an affected foetus, or carriers at risk of producing an affected offspring.

There is an increasing need for clinical geneticists to translate these fruits of basic research into health care. However, the number of clinical geneticists in the UK is very small and this is a matter of considerable concern; in consequence, the Medical

Research Council (MRC) earmarked fellowships and studentships in the area of clinical genetics to provide much needed training opportunities. This is an issue that needs to be addressed on a national level.

Data generated by genetics research is shared through national and international conferences and via publications. In addition, the MRC has organised a number of focused workshops designed to bring together experts from different disciplines (e.g. clinical geneticists with psychosocial experts and behaviouralists). Data generated by the global human genome project is uniquely deposited in public databases for the benefit of all.

2. Why is it worthwhile to map and sequence the human genome? What are the relative advantages of mapping expressed genes only versus completely sequencing the genome?

The human genome consists of some 3 million bases on twenty-four distinct chromosomes; it is believed these compose some 50,000–100,000 genes. The aim of the human genome programme is to locate the position of all the DNA and to decode the genetic information contained therein. This will of course include aberrant information present in disease genes. Strategies centre on construction of the genetic map, the physical map and ultimately the complete DNA sequence. The genetic map shows the relative positions of gene loci on the chromosomes and is derived from studies of inheritance. The physical map shows the identifiable landmarks (e.g. genes or markers) on DNA, regardless of inheritance. Sequencing is the ordering of nucleotides in a stretch of DNA, a gene, a chromosome or the entire genome.

Sequencing of the whole genome will reveal sequences with important functions that might otherwise go unidentified. Since only around 10 per cent of the bases are thought to contain useful information, some researchers have opted to sequence only the expressed genes; this approach offers short-term returns by avoiding gene poor regions; however, it has a number of inherent problems. Firstly, it is probably impossible to discover all the genes; secondly, the possibility of studying control sequences is denied; thirdly, complete sequences are not always easy to obtain for large genes; fourthly, sequencing costs will fall only in the context of large-scale genomic sequencing, and lastly there are problems in dealing with multigene families.

The MRC supports work using both strategies.

3. What will it tell us about the human species and the individual that would not otherwise accrue from piecemeal studies?

The human genome project is a task too great for any one country to succeed alone. One of the special features of genome research is the requirement for national and international collaboration. Different research groups work on specific levels of genome organisation. Co-ordination of these approaches can be further enhanced by combining the efforts of groups with specific technical expertise, so as to generate more multidisciplinary approaches. Further, as information emerges about the sequence and function of various genes, it must be assembled into a single up-to-the-minute picture which is available to all researchers. All this systematic effort will provide a complete understanding of the genetic basis of man. Piecemeal studies would not benefit from the co-ordinated approach that permits the significance of newly generated information to be appreciated in the broader context.

4. *To what extent are human characteristics determined by the genome and to what extent does the environment influence the expression of genes?*

Normal variations in human characteristics such as personality, intelligence and physique may be explained by the inheritance of multiple genes and their interaction together with environmental influences. Such genes do not determine personality or behaviour – there is little doubt that the social and psychological environments that envelop a child in his/her formative years are the most powerful influences on personality and future behaviour – but the genes can influence how a child reacts to its environment.

5. *How much is understood about the organisation of coding information in the genome? Is it conceivable that interventions such as those produced by gene therapy might have unforeseen effects?*

The human genome contains up to 3 million base pairs, but it is believed that only 10 per cent of these may contain useful information which is read out in blocks called exons; the exons are separated by DNA segments called introns whose function is presently unknown.

The aim of gene therapy is to make good a defective gene in the body cells where it is required, by providing the right genetic information, under proper control, in precisely those cells that need it for their normal function. Thus far it has been possible only to supplement a defective gene, not to replace it; neither is it yet possible to lodge a gene precisely where it would naturally be. In time it may be feasible to harness the natural process of recombination which allows formation of new combinations of genes. Legislation is in place to ensure that procedures are conducted at the highest practicable safety levels (e.g. Clothier Report[1] and the Gene Therapy Advisory Committee). . . .

8. *What has the UK's contribution been, absolutely and relative to other countries?*

It is widely recognised that the UK has a thoroughly credible national genome programme. One tangible measure of the UK's contribution comes from a bibliometric analysis conducted in 1990. This showed that whereas the US had 47 per cent of total publications in human genetic mapping, the UK contributed 12 per cent, France 6 per cent and other countries together 12 per cent; importantly, the UK had twice the number of entries recorded for any country other than the US. The combined European contribution was 31 per cent of the total, a figure which vastly exceeded that of Japan (6 per cent) and approached that of the US (47 per cent). We do not have more recent analyses. In terms of overall funding, UK support does not match that committed by the US or Japan.

A complementary programme to the MRC Human Genome Mapping Project is the MRC's initiative in the Genetic Approach to Human health, which aims to take the fruits of genome research into health care. This initiative has a broad remit, covering the analysis of disease loci to identify the mutations giving rise to particular genetic disorders, the enhancement of transgenic animal facilities, the molecular biological, biochemical and physiological characterisation of the gene products responsible for dysfunction and the development of therapeutic approaches based on the findings, the development of new tests for carriers and for embryo screening, the development of somatic gene therapy in animal models and for clinical use, studies on the psychological and social considerations surrounding the practice of genetic counselling and gene therapy, and evaluation of the benefits, costs and implementation strategies of transferring the new technologies into health service provision for prevention and treatment. This initiative commenced in 1992 and was allocated a budget for some £80 million over five years; this is not a ring-fenced initiative.

The MRC spends around £10 million per annum on underpinning genetics research.

9. *How does the Human Genome Mapping Project stimulate and benefit from comparable studies of other organisms of basic scientific, pharmaceutical and/or agricultural importance?*

To facilitate our understanding of human biology and disease it is essential to study a diverse range of model organisms whose genomes are less complicated. In spite of the differences, many genes fulfil similar basic functions. Hence our knowledge of gene function and mechanisms is underpinned by studies of yeast, plants, the fruit fly, the worm, the puffer fish, the mouse and farm animals. Strategies for mapping, sequencing and informatics are best developed first in these organisms because of their lower genetic complexity and ease of manipulation. In addition, the analysis of model systems has an intrinsic importance both in understanding the model organisms themselves and in industry and agriculture. Studies on the genomes of model organisms are being undertaken in parallel with human genome research to generate comparative data and to aid functional understanding of the human genome. Many of the basic features of genome organisation are universal and the assessment of experimentally induced alterations to sequenced regions of the genome can be undertaken only in model systems.

10. *How do genes make cells, make organs, make organisms?*

Genes carry the information that cells and organisms need to reproduce themselves. They are made of deoxyribonucleic acid (DNA), which consists of chains of four different types of nucleotides, abbreviated as A, T, G and C. Each of the forty-six chromosomes in the cells of the human body consists of two DNA molecules entwined as a double helix, each containing from 50 million to 250 million nucleotides. The A nucleotide of one DNA molecule is always associated with a T nucleotide of the other DNA molecule, and a C with a G. This 'complementarity' allows DNA molecules to be copied accurately.

Genes make proteins, and the sequence of the different nucleotides in a gene defines the sequence of amino-acids in the protein it encodes. These proteins have diverse functions. Some are required to control DNA replication. Others are structural components of the cell. Still others are enzymes, which process nutrients and allow the synthesis of other cellular constituents such as lipids and complex sugars. In multicellular organisms, different cells become specialised for different functions. Skin cells provide an impermeable barrier from the environment; muscle cells allow us to move; nerve cells are specialised for communication. Each of these specialised cell types expresses specific proteins. Skin cells make keratin, muscle cells contract because they make special types of myosin, and nerve cells make neurofilament proteins which extend along the length of axons and provide rigidity. Each of these specialised proteins is encoded by a specific gene. The process of embryonic development ensures that these different cell types, which express different proteins, form in the right number, in the right place and at the right time.

It is very important to understand how development is controlled and the UK in particular has made major advances in this field. Proteins have been identified which control the rate at which cells divide, and this provides insights into how the size of organs is controlled. We now know that cell–cell interactions are involved in specifying cell fate. For example, a protein secreted by one group of cells in an embryo can instruct neighbouring cells to form muscle. Great progress has been made in identifying these signalling proteins, and we now also understand how cells respond to these signalling molecules. In particular, it has been shown that these molecules can cause synthesis of new intracellular proteins to define a cell's position in the embryo, as well as defining what type of cell it should eventually become. These intracellular proteins include the so-called Hox proteins.

11. *What are the effects of malfunctions?*

Malfunctions in a gene may have many different effects, ranging from the catastrophic (the death of the embryo) to the relatively minor, to the invisible. The inactivation of a gene involved in cell replication may prevent the fertilised egg from dividing. Inactivation of a gene called Brachyury causes loss of posterior structures of the embryo. Inactivation of the Dystrophin gene causes Duchenne muscular dystrophy, and the gene has recently been identified which when mutated causes osteochondrodyplasia, a form of dwarfism. Finally, people who inherit from their parents only one functional copy of the p53 gene are predisposed to cancer.

12. *How frequently do new variations arise?*

Variants in a gene arise by mutation, which occurs when a mistake is made in DNA replication. The rate at which this occurs can only be estimated indirectly. In general, however, the fidelity of DNA replication is very high, and a single gene that encodes an average sized protein (containing 1,000 nucleotides) would suffer mutation only once in about a million cell generations. Mutations affect 1–2 per cent liveborn infants and cause about 8.5 per cent of child deaths and 7 per cent stillbirths and neonatal deaths.

EVOLUTION

13. *What evidence is there of continuing evolutionary change in humans?*

There is extensive evidence of continuing evolutionary change in humans. For example, the New World was populated some 25,000 years ago, but changes in the skin colour of populations of Central South America and the tip of South America have been recorded in the last 10,000 years. Moreover, it is believed that the malaria parasite evolved only 10,000 years ago.

14. *What may be the consequences of modern social organisation for human evolution?*

Modern social organisation is crucial to the future of human evolution. Humans are no longer a rare species and there are no longer the same opportunities for genetic drift. For example, tribal people in the Amazon living in different villages were genetically very distinct 1,000 years ago; this is no longer the case.

15. *What may the consequences of environmental change be for human evolution?*

The consequences of environmental change for human evolution are less than one might think. People are now able to manipulate the environment to suit themselves, so there are no longer the same pressures for human evolution. For example, in the case of diabetes, diets have been actively changed rather than simply leaving change to human evolution.

16. *What might be the evolutionary impact of selective fertilisation or termination and of other forms of extreme discrimination?*

Such effects are somewhat unpredictable. In the case of rare, persistent, harmful, dominant diseases (e.g. Huntington's chorea) selective fertilisation or termination is possible, but the scale on which this happens has low impact. For recessive disorders the impact is more unpredictable due to the effect of reproductive compensation (i.e., couples tend to have additional children to compensate for any lost through selective termination).

MEDICAL IMPLICATIONS

17. *What proportion of diseases stem from a single genetic defect? How many of these are currently diagnosed? What is the incidence in the UK population of known carriers and sufferers of each related disease and disability? How does this incidence in the UK vary from that in the world generally and how does it vary between groups in the UK? How does the research effort into particular genetic diseases correlate with their frequency?*

The proportion of diseases stemming from a single genetic defect is unknown because research is generating new knowledge all the time. The Department of Health should be consulted on the number of single gene diseases currently diagnosed and about the incidence of known carriers and sufferers in the UK and elsewhere. Research effort into particular genetic diseases does not necessarily correlate with their frequency; it relates more to the feasibility of the research (e.g. one Adenosine Deaminase Deficiency patient was able to be treated with gene therapy because the technology was available).

18. *What is the likely clinical impact of mapping susceptibility genes for common diseases? How far are we from being able to screen effectively for the genes which might predispose towards a wide range of diseases? What diseases are likely to be involved? What will the cost of such tests be?*

The clinical impact of mapping susceptibility genes for common diseases is likely to be very high, since better knowledge of genes and their products will lead to improvements in diagnosis, rational drug design and gene therapy. The ability to detect individuals who are carriers for specific gene defects will also facilitate epidemiological studies of the risks associated with environmental or occupational factors. In the past five years or so more than fifty new tests for genetic conditions have been developed; these include tests for well known genetic diseases such as muscular dystrophy and cystic fibrosis. Tests for common diseases such as cancer, hypertension, diabetes and heart disease are still under development. There have been numerous suggestions that the APOe4–Alzheimer association could be used to identify people at high risk; tests for allergies and osteoporosis are not inconceivable for the future.

The Department of Health may be able to advise about the likely cost of such tests.

19. *How much of genetic diagnosis is conducted as a routine medical service, and how much is associated with research programmes? Are some diseases with a known genetic cause not being diagnosed, and if so why not?*

Most diagnoses are probably conducted in a service manner, but are certainly not routine; pilot projects might, on the other hand, be considered as research. Scientific endeavour centres on the development of new or improved diagnostic tests.

Demand from families is an important factor in terms of which diseases are being diagnosed; the existence of an effective lay society also raises the profile of disease. On the other hand, the development of diagnostic tests for diseases where treatments are of limited effectiveness, or where no treatments are currently available, is unsatisfactory.

Education and counselling are vital components of the genetic testing process; MRC is funding research into these important issues.

20. *What proportion of diseases are expected to have some significant relation with particular genetic traits? How will the influences of nature and nurture on an individual's likely susceptibility to disease be determined?*

Almost all diseases will have some genetic component; this does not mean that there are not also very important environmental factors. The influences of nature and nurture may be investigated through studies of twins.

21. *How common is it for genes to have more than one function (e.g. the gene which controls sickle cell disease also offers protection against malaria)? How common is it for more than one gene to have the same function? What implications does this have for treatment?*

The different apparent effects of a genetic disease usually turn out to have some common pathway. The example given of sickle cell disease is not one of different function, but of the same alteration having effects that may be, on balance, helpful in one situation and harmful in another.

22. *Is it possible that changes in the coding of the genome such as those produced by gene therapy could have unforeseen effects?*

This has already been addressed as part of question 5. There will inevitably be some concerns that inserted genes may interfere with the function of another critical gene or activate an oncogene; however, the regulatory bodies scrutinise proposals for human gene therapy trials and permit only those that meet the agreed standards to go ahead.

23. *Though therapy is aimed at somatic cells, how is the germ line protected? Should it be?*

Whilst it is not possible to protect the germ line completely, efforts are always directed towards ensuring that somatic gene therapy is given locally and targeted to those specific cells that need to be treated. To verify that somatic gene therapy has not inadvertently affected offspring and successive generations, monitoring should extend at least into the next generation and, in so far as is possible, should continue over several generations.

In practice, germ line gene therapy where the new gene would be passed on to the next generation has been deemed to be illegal for the foreseeable future.

24. *What considerations lead to the introduction of human clinical trials of gene-based directed therapies? Is there . . . a possibility of conflict between the interests of the individual patient taking part in the trial and the wider group of those suffering from the disease? How is this managed? Will new clinical trials procedures need to be developed?*

The introduction of human clinical trials of gene-based directed therapies stems from the exciting possibility of being able to treat a genetic disease that cannot presently be treated in any other way, or where existing treatments are inadequate. The desirability of introducing one-shot gene therapy that will last a lifetime is no different in concept from the now historic aim of producing a one-shot vaccine.

The regulatory authorities that consider applications for the introduction of gene therapy trials are responsible for ensuring that safety, efficacy and ethical considerations are adequately addressed. . . .

The potential conflict between the interests of individual patients taking part in gene therapy trials and the wider group of those suffering from the disease is managed by ensuring that the individual is provided with all necessary information and is able to give fully informed consent. The situation is not in principle different from other forms of clinical trials.

Since the number of patients entering a gene therapy trial is inevitably very small (between two and nine per trial at present) special consideration has to be given, in designing trials, to data management and to gathering information across different trials in order to access all relevant data on best practice.

THE ETHICS OF RESEARCH

25. *To what extent should geneticists be free to decide the parameters of their research? What influences their choices? What are the social implications of this research; is there a danger that genetic research will lead to a crudely deterministic view of human behaviour?*

Research involving human subjects or information about them requires Local Research Ethics Committee (LREC) approval (set up under Department of Health guidelines with lay input). It is important that research should continue even if the most obvious practical use is not currently acceptable, since the research may lead to other insights (e.g. basic research on embryos may lead to the feasibility of removal of embryos in cancer patients undergoing whole body therapy and their subsequent replacement).

Research choices are influenced by quality of life potential, wealth creation potential, understanding of human biology, and the feasibility of the research.

Genetics differs from most biology in that information gained about an individual has implications for their family; hence conventional ethical concepts relating to the individual need to be modulated. The MRC recognises and funds important research on environmental effects. Most geneticists are acutely aware that genes act only in an environmental context, never in isolation. There is no evidence currently of crude determinism; vigilance and efforts to increase public understanding should go hand in hand with genetics research.

26. *What is the current policy of the MRC and other research funding councils with regard to the ethical and social effects of research in genetics?*

The MRC seeks to ensure that awareness of potential users is promulgated on the basis of scientific facts and to support research on potential uses related to improving health. For example, research into genetics counselling and into psychosocial and behavioural studies falls squarely within the remit of the Council's Genetic Approach to Human Health Initiative; funding is also provided for training and for workshops that bring together scientists from different disciplines (e.g. psychologists and behaviouralists with clinical geneticists). The MRC takes account of the needs of users (including the public) in formulating its research strategy. MRC scientists are encouraged to convey to the public, through the media, through schools liaison, open days and science festivals the basis for and importance of MRC-funded work in genetics.

The other research councils should be consulted about their own policies.

THE ETHICS OF SCREENING AND TREATMENT

27. *What do we need to know about the ways in which genes work in order to make decisions about the use or regulation of genetic information? Are we likely to obtain that information?*

It will be important to know whether particular sequences are becoming unstable, how often sequences become mutagenised, and how often mutagenesis leads to new targets. There is much information available already from animal experiments (e.g. on the fruit fly *Drosophila*) but more data are required; such needs can be satisfied only through further research.

The exact use to which genetic information is put is very important. For example, we must be very sure that DNA fingerprinting is reliable when used for convictions or for paternity suits; reproductive choice, on the other hand, may only need a probability range for the chance of bearing an affected offspring. Conventional considerations, such as false positive and false negative, are also important, as is variation in the severity of disease, and the population base used for probability (e.g. in the context of fingerprinting). In terms of gene therapy there are many other considerations (e.g. the target cells, regulation of gene expression, etc.).

Genetic information has already found a number of successful applications: for example, genetic fingerprinting and virtual eradication of thalassaemia from the Cypriot population via screening programmes.

Valuable lessons may be learned from experience with AIDS about the ways to handle information in relation to insurance, etc.

28. *How are human reproductive technologies regulated in the UK? How does this compare with regulation in other countries?*

This question is more properly addressed by the Department of Health, but a few notes follow:

(i) *Technologies to assist fertility.* Drugs are regulated by the Medicines Control Agency (MCA) and *in vitro* fertilisation by the Human Fertilisation and Embryology Authority (HFEA).

(ii) *Technologies to prevent unwanted pregnancies.* Pre-conception: drugs are regulated by the MCA. For other devices, the EU is introducing similar regulations to those for drugs. Post-conception: drugs are regulated by the MCA. Clinicians are regulated by the General Medical Council.

(iii) *Technologies to select against unwanted characteristics.* Carrier diagnosis is through regulation of the clinical profession (General Medical Council), as is post-implantation diagnosis; pre-implantation diagnosis is regulated by the HFEA as part of IVF.

The Department of Health should be consulted about regulations in other countries.

29. *Are there ethical problems about gene therapy, either somatic or germ line? If so, what are these? In what way does manipulation of the germ line in the laboratory differ from natural variation?*

The first question is well covered by the Clothier report. Somatic gene therapy is essentially equivalent to transplantation. There is a need for safety considerations (e.g. not delivering to the germ line) and the source of the gene may worry some people. Germ line gene therapy is potentially a better solution, but since it affects the next generation there is a greater obligation for safety. However, this is also true for many conventional treatments (e.g. cytotoxic drugs for cancer patients). The situation *vis-à-vis* germ line gene therapy needs to be reviewed in due course in the light of experience with somatic gene therapy.

Natural variation involves three processes: (1) there is one chromosome pair in each parent. At random the progeny will inherit, from each parent, one of the two chromosomes in each pair; (2) rare recombination events leading to new combinations of DNA on one chromosome; (3) rarer mutations leading to a modified gene.

Laboratory manipulation can involve all these, but typically specifically seeks to focus on recombination to insert the normal form of the disease gene. In the laboratory it is possible to introduce genes from different species not limited by conventional hybrid non-viability/sterility.

Experimental manipulation of the germ line which introduces mutations in a non-targeted and small-scale way will not be different from mutations that occur through natural variation. Significant effects on the germ line would be generated only by large-scale manipulations (e.g. those involving all patients and carriers of a particular genetic disease world-wide). However, natural variation is an on-going process and it is often the case that as soon as one disease is eradicated from the global population it is replaced by another (e.g. polio and AIDS).

Trials of gene therapy in patients are just beginning. Success will depend in part upon acceptability both to the public and to those eligible for trials. This in turn will depend on the quality of the information provided in the public arena and in the clinical setting.

NOTES

This chapter originated as a memorandum submitted in evidence to the House of Commons Science and Technology Committee in 1994 by the Medical Research Council. It is reprinted (with abridgements) by permission of HMSO from vol. 4 of the committee's report, *Human Genetics: the Science and its Consequences* (London: HMSO, 1995).

1 *Report of the Committee on the Ethics of Gene Therapy*, CM 1788, London, HMSO (1991).

4

GENETICS AND INSURANCE

Sheila A. M. McLean and Philippa Gannon

There can be little doubt that the newest weapon in medicine's armory – the rapid development in genetic knowledge – has had, and will continue to have, a profound impact on humanity. As the knowledge grows exponentially, it is equally certain that every citizen will have cause to evaluate its impact on him or herself. The so-called genetic revolution will fuel reappraisal of conventional medicine, will raise complex and subtle ethical problems at both a personal and a community level and will challenge the law to make a sophisticated response.

INTRODUCTION

The capacity to identify the genetic component in disease entities and behavioural characteristics will serve to distinguish each individual from the other, whilst at the same time – since genes are shared – identifying common characteristics which bind people together. The inexplicable will become explicable; the unknown known. Evidently, our increasing capacities do not exist or grow in a vacuum, and the extent to which this knowledge works for good or bad will, in large part, be predicated on the value systems which are used to underpin our treatment of it. Even if it were plausible to argue that knowledge is inherently value-free, it undoubtedly has the potential to become intensely value-laden when it is sought to turn theory into practice.

The intimate knowledge which can now be gained of people's propensities to behavioural or clinical characteristics is of interest not just to the individual but also to the society of which s/he is a part. As the Danish Council of Ethics[1] put it: 'the completely new information and scope for action destined to follow from the

87

mapping of the human genome will alter fundamental ethical concepts such as autonomy, integrity, privacy, quality of life and so on.'[2] Interest in this information may come from a variety of sources – the family, the state, employers and, of course, the insurance industry. Although tensions exist in each of these areas, perhaps they are most acutely observed in the attempt to balance the interest of the individual in the privacy of health-related information and that of the insurance industry in continuing to provide a service which is economically viable for them.

Chadwick and Ngwena[3] describe the nature of insurance in this way:

> The essence of an insurance contract, whether it be health, life or otherwise, is that in return for the insured's premium, the insurer agrees to assume the risk of an uncertain event in which the insured has an interest and undertakes to pay a benefit, in cash or in kind, if the event occurs.[4]

Or, to put it another way:

> Insurance of all types is based on the complementary principles of solidarity and equity in the face of uncertain risks. In insurance, solidarity has been taken to imply the sharing by the population, as a whole or in broad groups, of benefits and costs; while equity has been taken to imply that the contribution of individuals should be approximately in line with their known level of risk.[5]

Genetic knowledge, however, has the capacity to modify, if not fundamentally alter, the balance between these latter two principles. Self-evidently, the insurance industry wishes to continue issuing policies, but equally obviously it will also wish to minimise risk. Thus the more clearly individual risks can be identified the more critical they will become in the underwriting process. As has been noted,

> Insurers argue that they do not want to decrease their business by excluding large numbers of people from coverage. . . . Factors are presently not favourable to the use of genetic testing by insurance companies, but participants expect these factors to change. . . . Improved understanding among underwriters could reduce the number of baseless

rejections of people unlikely to fall ill or die prematurely, but individuals who carry detectable genetic risks could still be rejected or charged higher premiums according to the definition of fairness used by the insurance industry.[6]

Moreover, individuals who currently subsidise the risks taken by others may have an interest in targeting specific risk-related characteristics or behaviour, in order that they may ultimately be given preferential treatment in terms of premiums. And, of course, those who turn out not to have been favoured by the genetic dice may wish to claim a strong privacy interest in information which might result in their being disadvantaged in insurance, either through elevated premiums or through outright refusal of cover.

Before looking in more depth at the issues raised by the new genetics it is worth making one point. Anything that is said about controlling and monitoring the use of genetic information could, at least in part, be applied to other health-related data. As the US Insurance Task Force noted, 'The standard personal medical history . . . is a rich source of genetic information.'[7] leading it to conclude that '[p]olicies intended to protect genetic privacy will need to address the privacy of health-related knowledge in general'.[8]

GENETIC INFORMATION AND PRIVACY

One critical impact of genetics, however, will be fundamentally to reshape the debate about privacy in health matters. Traditionally, this has been founded on the relatively uncontroversial application of two values – confidentiality and secrecy. With limited exceptions, for example in the case of infectious diseases, people have been free to expect that health-related information will be maintained in confidence by their clinician, and have been able to draw a public veil over their own health status. But genetic information is different on several grounds, leading to the conclusion that these seemingly complementary and all-encompassing principles may be insufficient or inappropriate in the future.

It has been estimated that '[g]enetic and pre-genetic diseases affect one in every twenty people by the age of 25 and perhaps as many as two in three people during their lifetime'.[9] Although not everyone will suffer in any way as a result of this, it is clear that the pervasive nature of genetic conditions will mean that everyone will have to contemplate the possibility that their genes will affect their life in ways more dramatic than was previously known. The nature/ nurture debate has been revived and new life breathed into it by the inexorable search to complete the mapping of the human genome, leading to human beings being 'genetically laid bare and vulnerable as never before'.[10]

It would, of course, be wrong to paint a totally black picture. Genetic knowledge will undoubtedly lead to huge benefits. The possibility of disease identification will lead to the search for, and hopefully the discovery of, therapies and cures. The shape of human health in the next century will doubtless be significantly informed by what we now know and what we will discover.[11] However, it is not inappropriate also to sound a note of caution. The simple presumption that the identification or eradication of disease will stand alone as a 'good' thing is not one which can necessarily be made. In the same way as traditional diagnoses have influenced the lives of some people, so too our health status in the future will not become any less of a social, political or economic factor merely because it is described in a different, more scientifically sophisticated way.

One example of this relates directly to the subject of this chapter – the relationship between the insurance industry and the potential insured. The insurance industry plays a powerful and critical role in most societies. Although the subject matter of an insurance contract may vary, the ultimate purpose of any contract of insurance is to assess and underwrite the costs – personal or economic – of unexpected hazards or risks. As a social phenomenon, then, insurance fulfils two purposes. First, it acts as a threshold device to determine the ability of an individual to enter into other contracts. For example, in the UK most mortgage companies require an individual to obtain a life insurance policy before money will be provided in order to purchase property. Second, insurance is increasingly used to supplement public services, for example by the purchasing of private health care policies or private pension schemes. Different kinds of contract may raise different kinds of issues, but we will proceed from the perspective that the central questions are about values which underpin all insurance, no matter which area of life it is designed to cover. The critical matters relate not to the specifics of a particular contract but rather to the principles which demonstrate and define the potential for conflict between the interests of the industry and the interests of the individual.

The point has already been made that genetic information shares characteristics with other health-related information. However, it also goes beyond this. Genetic information can be distinguished from other health-related information on a number of grounds. First, genetic information may be predictive rather than descriptive. That is, the possibility of disease can be tested for and identified when an individual is asymptomatic, leading to an expansion in the period of time during which an individual may categorise him- or herself as a patient, with all the consequences which flow from that.[12] Second, genetic information is of direct relevance to other members of the individual's family, making the arguments from secrecy and confidentiality potentially more difficult to sustain. Third, our capacity to make genetic diagnoses far exceeds our capacity to do anything about them.[13] Thus, even accepting that there are non-genetic disorders which also fit this category, the diagnosis of a genetic disorder is considerably less likely to bring with it the prospect of prevention, palliation or cure. That being so, there are powerful arguments that people have a right not to know their genetic make-up.

Although the tradition of modern medical ethics has been to develop a right to *know* information, the genetic revolution has seen the embryonic development of claims that there should also be a right *not* to know. This claim is in part influenced by the therapeutic shortfall already referred to, but it is also based on the possibility of discrimination which is inherent in certain kinds of information, such as genetic information.[14] In the context of insurance, it is this fear of being forced to acquire potentially devastating information without hope of cure and then being required to divulge it to others who may use it to our prejudice that is most acute. For example, a *Time*/CNN poll reported in *Time* magazine in 1994 found that 'Of those polled, 90 per cent said they thought it should be against the law for insurance companies to use genetic tests to decide whom to insure.'[15]

There are two important issues surrounding genetic information which will be considered here. First, there is the question of obtaining information. This question particularly is concerned with the manner in which the relevant data are come by. Second, there are issues to be considered concerning the use to which it is subsequently put.

For the insurance industry, the more information which it can accumulate about a potential insured, the more accurate – in theory at least – will be its assessment of risk and the more appropriate will be the premium demanded. No longer would it be necessary to cover blanket groups – rather, the individual's risk category can be assessed on an informed calculation of the risk run by that particular person. The insurance industry, therefore, will benefit from minimising the chance associated with insurance (at least as far as genetic predisposition is concerned) and may be able to favour others who do not have such predispositions.

Even if such a highly individualised approach is neither possible nor practical the industry can still argue that better and fuller information is merely an extension of the data which they already use to assess premiums, and that the drive to acquire it is in no way more controversial than the current practices of the industry. Thus the driver with a bad history of accidents will, apparently uncontroversially, be expected to pay higher premiums for motor vehicle insurance; the smoker will expect to pay higher life insurance premiums, and the diabetic may be asked for higher premiums for health insurance. Thus it might be asked, since insurance plays an increasingly important social role, and the survival of the industry therefore is of value, would it not be reasonable that the industry should obtain such knowledge? There are, in reality, two questions here. The first relates to the value of the information itself and the second to the means of acquiring it.

If, as seems entirely plausible, a person's genetic make-up will affect quality or length of life, then it is self-evident that the insurer will have a legitimate interest in knowing it. Indeed, failure to disclose known or reasonably knowable health-related information would render any policy taken out null and void. The contract of insurance is one of *uberrima fides*, requiring that the potential insured notifies the potential insurer of all known factors which might affect the decision whether or not to enter into a legal contract. In effect, the person who knows (or should reasonably know) of genetic predisposition has no practical option but to inform the insurance company. There would be little logic in paying premiums over a period of years in the certain knowledge that the policy would ultimately be invalidated.

PUBLICITY AND COERCION

However, if the capacity of the insurance industry to make accurate calculations is the ultimate value, and if genetic information can be made available, it is but a short step (and a logical one) to suggest that such information *should* be sought. In other words, the argument which supports full disclosure is also an argument which could be used to *require* information to be found out. Coercion in such matters, however, should be resisted, in the same way as controversy surrounds any suggestion that people should be forced to find out their HIV status. As Schmidtke says:

> No matter what way a person comes to terms with such information – which may be either a blessing or be terrifying – in all societies where maximum priority is attached to the right to self-determination with regard to information there is a consensus that the decision for or against such predictive diagnostics and the result thereof must remain a private matter.[16]

Forcing individuals to acquire evidence of their genetic status would, therefore, fly directly in the face of the claim that people have a right not to know about their genetic (or indeed other) status. Herein lies the first, and arguably the most profound, of the tensions between individual and industry. The only way in which the industry can find out the information it claims a legitimate interest in is if the individual *is* tested and thereby acquires that information to pass on. For the individual who does not wish to know his or her own genetic status, this could be profoundly distressing.

Yet, although mandatory testing is not yet contemplated within insurance circles, it is obviously the only way of providing the full picture which the logic of the argument would suggest the insurance industry – and other policyholders – would benefit from.

For the moment, then, the individual is at liberty to seek or not to seek genetic information, but once it is known it must be honestly disclosed to the insurers, otherwise any policy agreed upon will be invalid. The freedom not to seek information is highly valued, since many fear that a 'bad' result will result in their being refused insurance, or at least in elevating premiums. This highlights the second matter raised above – namely, what is done with the information once it is obtained. Two questions also arise here. First, is the information used appropriately; second, will its use result in discriminatory practices?

MISUSE OF GENETIC INFORMATION

There is reason for some concern that genetic information may be poorly understood and therefore inappropriately used. To an extent this fear may well be minimised in the UK by the Association of British Insurers' decision to appoint an independent genetics adviser, but it is implausible that such an appointment could meet every eventuality in the issuing of every policy. Assessment of genetic information, therefore, will still commonly be left in the hands of those trained in underwriting rather than in the hands of those trained in molecular biology, leaving wide open the possibility of misunderstanding. Just as with other health-related information, the presence of a particular gene does not predict with certainty the timing or severity of the onset of the linked condition, nor can it definitively answer the question whether or not death or additional health care costs will be the result of that genetic predisposition. Yet the aura of scientific certainty which pervades much of the discourse on genetics may lead the unwary or the ignorant into weighing genetic evidence more heavily in the decision-making scales than is actually merited. People may, therefore, be unfairly denied access to insurance or at least find that they enter the market at a significant financial disadvantage.

So the question of the use to which genetic information is put takes on considerable significance. The possibility that discriminatory practices will result from the identification of those with a propensity to certain conditions is one which cannot be discounted. Genetic discrimination is a feature of our recent past as well as of our predictable future.[17] Although likely to present in a much more sophisticated form than the pogroms of Nazi Germany or the forced sterilisation programmes of the US, the lives of individuals may yet be disvalued because of their genetic inheritance. Refusal of insurance would, given its significance to people in many aspects of their lives, be a significant social and economic handicap. It is already known that 'Americans are losing their jobs and health insurance based on information uncovered in genetic screens.'[18] Although genetic information may be relevant in some ways to employment and insurance practices, and therefore its use is not inevitably discriminatory, the points already made about the lack of understanding of what genetic test results actually tell us lead to the very real fear that its use will in fact be discriminatory rather than appropriate. And whilst loading premiums is currently an accepted practice, it must be remembered that it may be described as a relevant use of information rather than discrimination pure and simple.

GENETICS AND INSURANCE PRACTICE

These concerns are not the sole province of the academic. In 1995 the House of Commons Committee on Science and Technology[19] produced a report covering the entire spectrum of issues actually or potentially raised by the genetic revolution. The committee paid particular attention to the use of genetic information, expressing the general concern that 'genetic discrimination may happen inadvertently, and should be prevented'.[20] In its view, the real issues centred on the question of privacy, although it conceded that in employment and insurance third parties might wish to use information about genetic predisposition.[21] Witnesses giving evidence to the committee expressed concern about this, pointing to the potential for discrimination inherent in the use of information which is occasionally uncertain and sometimes poorly understood.

However, the evidence from the insurance industry itself was also significant. Earlier calls by the Nuffield Council on Bioethics[22] for a moratorium on the use of genetic information in insurance policies were resisted by the industry, not least because of the fear of adverse selection. The fear is that, if people are not required to disclose relevant information when they are taking out a policy, those who know themselves to have a high risk of developing a particular condition will insure themselves for substantial sums of money, whilst those who know themselves to be a good risk may be discouraged from taking out certain kinds of policy at all, thus skewing the insurance picture. Although this fear must be taken seriously, Chadwick and Ngwena point out that 'There is . . . no convincing evidence to suggest that insurers will be inundated with applicants who know that they constitute a high risk: not least because insurers already have in place contractually in-built methods for avoiding adverse selection.'[23] As has already been noted, these methods relate to the nature of the contract itself and would render the policy void in any event.

The view of the Science and Technology Committee was that the Association of British Insurers had not taken sufficient account of the possible problems which may arise from the impact of genetics on the industry and on the individuals concerned.[24] Its approach was described by the committee as one of 'undue complacency'.[25] In light of this, the committee recommended that the insurance industry should be given a year in which to come up with an acceptable solution, failing which legislation might be necessary.[26] In fact the industry took rather longer than that but did issue a policy statement in respect of life insurance for mortgages in February 1997.[27]

To an extent, its response may still be described as relatively sanguine. Noting that, in life insurance, 'around 95 per cent of all applicants are provided with insurance on standard terms and conditions . . .'[28] and that less than 1 per cent of applicants are refused cover, they present a picture which may suggest that the fears expressed above are overstated. However, these figures relate to past practices and do not take account of the extent to which genetics may impinge on insurance in the future. This is not to say that the industry has not taken the question seriously; the appointment of both a genetics adviser and an ethics committee shows that real consideration of potential difficulties is taking place.

For the moment, the life insurance members of the Association of British Insurers have concluded as follows:

> They will continue not to ask people to take genetic tests when applying for life insurance.
>
> For new applications for life insurance of up to a total of £100,000, which are directly linked to a new mortgage for a private dwelling being acquired for occupation by the live/ lives [sic] to be insured, the results of any genetic tests will not be taken into account by the insurance company if they are to the detriment of the applicant. As at present, account will continue to be taken of family history and of other medical information.
>
> For new applications for other life insurance policies, individual companies will decide whether or not they wish to take account of the results of genetic tests previously taken.[29]

Thus some concessions have been made to the privacy of genetic data, but clearly these are fairly limited. Large numbers of people may still find that they are expected to provide information and that it may be used to increase premiums or even deny them cover.

It would, of course, be naive and probably unfair to suggest that insurers should have no access to this kind of information whilst still allowing them to use other evidence associated with individual risk. The challenge, however, is to strike a balance between the interests at stake, a balance which the ABI's policy still leaves uncertain. This is because genetic information is different from other kinds of information. The usual consequences of personal ill health are substantially borne by the individual him- or herself. Genetic predisposition, however, potentially affects those within the immediate family group also. Not only does this postulate complex ethical or moral dilemmas for the unfortunate individual who discovers a serious genetic problem, in terms of, for example, whether or not to disclose the information to relatives, it also may result in family members being provided with facts about their possible health status which they would prefer not to have. *Their* right not to know becomes compromised.

THE IMPORTANCE OF INSURANCE

It is clear that the genetic revolution poses many problems for the individual in his or her interaction with the community of which he or she is a part. It may be thought that these general problems are of sufficient weight to render the question of access to insurance relatively unimportant. That, however, would be fundamentally to misunderstand the significance of insurance in contemporary Western society. As we have said, insurance which is no longer the prerogative of the rich; rather it is a prerequisite of full engagement in the community. Indeed, the maintenance of a thriving industry might well be seen as satisfying the public interest. Indeed, the public interest is also a consideration often used to justify a derogation from otherwise strict rules. For example, the obligation of confidentiality owed by doctor to patient is subject to an exception where disclosure is thought to be in the public interest.

However, this exception is ill defined. As Ngwena and Chadwick point out, '[it] is apparent from decided cases that the public interest exception can be invoked to protect an open rather than a closed category of interests. . . .'[30] Given the concerns already expressed, it is wise to be cautious before presuming that a case can be made in the public interest that the insurance industry has special interests which would mandate the breaching of other rights and interests which have traditionally had priority. In addition, any suggestion that information once gained must always be disclosed might act against the public interest by deterring people from undergoing genetic tests, particularly where the condition identified is (as many genetic conditions are) polyfactorial or influenced by environment as well as genes.

It is vital that a resolution of the tensions between the interest of the individual in privacy and in obtaining affordable insurance and the industry's legitimate desire for commercial viability is found sooner rather than later. Half-hearted *ad hoc* arrangements will do little to achieve this goal. The issues which must be addressed relate first to the voluntariness of obtaining information. It is anathema that people should be coerced into finding out information which they would otherwise wish not to know, with the possible exception of situations where failure to do so puts others at significant risk. Although genetic information affects more than the individual undergoing the test it is difficult to see how it could plausibly be argued that failure to know poses such a threat to others.

However, if it were to be assumed that the insurance industry (and/or existing policyholders) would indeed suffer dramatically were people allowed this right not to know, then there is a real danger that – uniquely – people could be forced to undergo testing or screening, with the intention that the information gained would be used to their detriment, or – probably less likely – in their favour. Those who would be favoured might see no objection, but the objection lies not in the satisfaction of the individual's desire for better treatment but rather in the invasion of fundamentally valuable principles. As has been said:

> The routine availability of identifiable genetic information about individuals may have effects that reach far beyond the provision of medical care. As the amount of detailed genetic information grows, society may be required to re-examine the basic principles of health and life insurance, review the rules that govern employment and hiring, reconsider the confidentiality rules that are part of the doctor–patient relationship, and in general reassess the way in which individuals are categorised and treated in a variety of social and economic relationships.[31]

Second, the insurance industry must seek to avoid discrimination in two ways. First, if people are not to be discouraged from seeking genetic information which may assist them in maintaining good levels of health, the industry must demonstrate its capacity to handle the information appropriately and in a balanced manner. Also, the approach of the industry to genetic information must be one which reflects values wider than the economic. Values such as formal justice and non-discrimination must underpin their use of such data.

These are significant challenges, but they must be resolved. The imminent completion of the Human Genome Project leads to the conclusion that appropriate value systems must be in place sooner rather than later. As the Danish Council of Ethics puts it:

it can be said that a decisive stand on the new challenges must be based on a choice between the two overall approaches: the utilitarian view or the approach based on the help motive and respect for the individual. The question, in other words is: must the principle purpose of applying human genetics be formulated in terms of the gain for the common good or in terms of the individual?[32]

NOTES

1 Danish Council of Ethics, *Ethics and Mapping of the Human Genome*, Copenhagen, 1993.
2 At p. 63.
3 R. Chadwick and C. Ngwena, 'The Human Genome Project, predictive testing and insurance contracts: ethical and legal responses', *Res Publica* 1, No. 2 (1995), 115.
4 At p. 118.
5 Nuffield Council on Bioethics, *Genetic Screening: Ethical Issues*, London, 1993, at p. 66, para. 7.6.
6 *Human Genome News* 4, No. 1 (May 1992), 5, at p. 6.
7 *Human Genome News* 5, No. 2 (July 1993), 1.
8 Ibid.
9 British Medical Association, *Our Genetic Future: The Science and Ethics of Genetic Technology*, Oxford, Oxford University Press, 1992, at p. 1.
10 J. C. Fletcher and D. C. Wertz, 'An international code of ethics in medical genetics before the human genome is mapped', in Z. Bankowski and A. Caprin (eds), *Genetics, Ethics and Human Values: Human Genome Mapping, Genetic Screening and Therapy*, Proceedings of the Twenty-fourth CIOMS Round Table Conference (held in Tokyo and Inuyama City, Japan, 22–27 July 1990), at p. 97.
11 As has been said, 'The new genetical anatomy will transform medicine and mitigate suffering in the twenty-first century.' T. Wilkie, *Perilous Knowledge: The Human Genome Project and its Implications*, London, Faber, 1993, at p. 1.
12 The Danish Council of Ethics (*Ethics and Mapping*, at p. 60) makes a telling point on this matter: 'Just as persons found through screening to have a particular gene or chromosome composition may happen to feel abnormal or outright ill . . . so may others react to the persons involved by giving them a wide berth.'

13 Cf. T. Friedmann, 'Opinion: the Human Genome Project – some implications of extensive "reverse genetic" medicine', *American Journal of Human Genetics* 46 (1990), 408, at p. 411: 'there remains a serious gap between disease characterization and treatment'.

14 Cf. J. Maddox, 'The case for the human genome', *Nature* 352 (4 July 1991), 11, at p. 11: 'The ethical objections to the sequencing of the human genome are necessarily more subtle. They range from the assertion that it would be improper that knowledge won in a scientific project such as this should be used to discriminate in novel ways between people seeking insurance cover or jobs, to the generalized alarm occasioned by any suggestion that eugenic improvement may be feasible. . . .'

15 P. Elmer-Dewitt, 'The genetic revolution', *Time*, 17 January 1994, No. 3, 34.

16 J. Schmidtke, 'Who owns the human genome? Ethical and legal aspects', *Journal of Pharmacy and Pharmacology* 44 (Suppl. 1), 205, at p. 208.

17 For discussion see S. A. M. McLean, 'The right to reproduce', in T. Campbell, S. McLean, D. Goldberg, T. Mullen (eds), *Human Rights: From Rhetoric to Reality*, Oxford, Blackwell, 1988.

18 Elmer-Dewitt, 'The genetic revolution', at p. 39.

19 House of Commons Science and Technology Committee, *Human Genetics: The Science and its Consequences*, Session 1994–5, London, HMSO.

20 Ibid., para. 221.

21 Ibid., para. 224.

22 Nuffield Council on Bioethics, *Genetic Screening*.

23 Chadwick and Ngwena, 'The Human Genome Project', at p. 119.

24 House of Commons Science and Technology Committee, *Human Genetics*, at para. 247.

25 Ibid.

26 House of Commons Science and Technology Committee, *Human Genetics*, at para. 248.

27 Association of British Insurers, *Life Insurance and Genetics: A Policy Statement*, London, February 1997.

28 Association of British Insurers, 'Life Insurance and Genetics' (information sheet), London, February 1997.

29 Association of British Insurers, *Policy Statement*.

30 C. Ngwena and R. Chadwick, 'Genetic diagnostic information and the duty of confidentiality: ethics and law', *Medical Law International* 1 (1993), No. 73, at p. 81.

31 US Congress, House of Representatives, Committee on Government Operations, *Designing Genetic Information Policy: The Need for an Independent Policy Review of the Ethical, Legal and Social Implications of the Human Genome Project*, Washington, D.C., Government Printing Office, 1992, at p. 2.

32 Danish Council of Ethics, *Ethics and Mapping*, at p. 64.

5

HIV AND INSURANCE

Heather Draper

In the late 1980s the insurance industry responded to forecasts of an HIV epidemic by loading the premiums of single men seeking life insurance and by revising their proposal questionnaires to include questions designed to assess the risk of the applicant contracting HIV disease. These measures were justified by appealing to the nature of the insurance industry and warnings from government actuaries of a potential explosion in claims from AIDS-related deaths. The industry argued that it was increasing the premiums of those who were thought at the time to be most at risk, and that it was standard practice to load premiums for high-risk groups and to refuse insurance to applicants likely to make substantial claims in the near future. It would be unacceptable, they argued, to those at low risk (e.g. married couples) to subsidise high-risk groups (e.g. single men). Tales about unscrupulous clients increasing insurance cover after they had found out they were HIV positive were cited as evidence of the need to be vigilant.

In answer to claims that this practice was unfair to those who were excluded from affordable insurance, the industry responded that it *was* fair under the principles of insurance and that, what is more, it was not the industry's responsibility to provide social welfare and health services for everyone. The industry's obligation was to provide insurance services with a view to making a profit for shareholders.

Whilst insurers are justified in estimating the level of risk they are being asked to take on, the methods used to assess risk can be dubious. Likewise, whilst it may be legitimate for the insurance industry to claim that it exists to make a profit rather than to provide vital services, that does not absolve it of all responsibility to those at most risk of contracting HIV. This chapter will look at how the obligation to provide insurance may depend on market size, monopoly and 'captive' markets. It will also look at good practice in assessing risk and settling claims. Finally, it will highlight some of the potential problems in relation to HIV to be found in Permanent Health Insurance (PHI) and Critical Illness Insurance (CII) policies.

PUBLIC *V.* PRIVATE HEALTH INSURANCE

In some countries, health services are provided by the state from taxation. Although such services may be less comprehensive in practice than in theory, they do often sustain a network of public hospitals and primary care facilities. Where such services exist, private health care is not vital as a means of obtaining good health care. In the UK, for instance, no one who is HIV positive or who has gone on to develop AIDS has to find resources for health care and no one is left without any health cover at all.[1] At worst one is likely to be left with less choice about the timing of consultations and a longer wait for non-urgent services. Commercial health cover is often seen as a means of enabling those who can afford to do so to obtain some services – usually elective or non-urgent services – quickly or at a time of their own choosing. The advantages of having this cover are not necessarily great. Many of those who have private health insurance see the same doctors in the same hospitals as NHS patients. If they discover that they have a previously undetected chronic illness, their private insurance will usually pay for treatment only for a limited time: in the UK, at least, policies have to be renewed frequently, and chronic conditions are unlikely to go on being insured after renewal, as they then count as pre-existing conditions which are excluded from cover. So even if someone who already had private health insurance contracted HIV disease after taking out a policy, it would have very little impact on any long-term care they needed, especially as they would probably not have treatable symptoms until after the relevant cover had lapsed.

What about those who are HIV positive in places where private health care insurance is the only means of gaining access to decent health care? Clearly the consequences of refusal of insurance are very much more serious. Does that fact by itself constrain private insurers not to refuse insurance applications from people at risk of contracting HIV disease? Well, it certainly has *some* moral weight. How much weight will depend on at least two factors: how big the risk of contracting HIV is; and what the money amount of the coverage is. The smaller the risk and the smaller the money amount of the coverage, the bigger the obligation on the insurer to take the risk. In certain market conditions the obligation to accept even high-value policy applications may be considerable. To see this, it is important to be clear about the position of private health insurers in the absence of compulsory state insurance schemes. At least in the developed world, insurers in such environments often have access to a large pool of reasonably wealthy, reasonably healthy, reasonably young applicants for insurance who, if they are prudent, will take out insurance, and who often have it taken out for them through employers' group insurance schemes. There is no reason why the health insurance business in such environments should not be profitable even if some applicants at high risk of contracting HIV disease are sold policies on standard terms. Again, there is no reason why the the health insurance business should not remain profitable if lots of people at medium risk of contracting HIV disease are sold policies at higher premiums. And there is probably even room (see below) for schemes that sell the very high-risk very expensive policies for insurance up to a certain substantial amount. The scope for profitability that results from a big market for something most people think they need and are willing to pay for is itself a reason, in addition to the moral reason provided by the consequences of refusal, for selling even large policies to those at some risk of contracting HIV disease.

CAPTIVE *V.* QUASI-CAPTIVE MARKETS

Background market conditions affect the strength of the moral obligation we have been considering. Where commercial insurance operates alongside compulsory state insurance (national insurance), it has to compete for the business of those who already pay for health cover through taxation, and for whom additional cover is a desirable luxury rather than a necessity. Competition itself can lead insurance companies to take calculated risks, but it is not unreasonable for companies to be cautious about the insurance applications they accept, as the market is likely to be small to begin with. When the market is very large because of the absence of a state scheme, the chances are good of individual companies getting a pool of risks that keeps them in profit and provides the ill with good treatment, without punitive rates for those at somewhat higher than normal risk of serious illness. If it is commercially possible to include the higher risk in the pool, and if it is morally awful for them to be excluded, there is no moral reason for not including them. This reasoning increases in force when the market is made maximally big by legislation that *forces* everyone with the means of buying insurance to do so. In such circumstances there is a *captive market* (on analogy with a 'captive audience') for health insurance and so a corresponding obligation on the insurance industry to take on risk up to the level where doing so threatens the existence of the market by wiping out profit or wiping out all competition.

I am not arguing that relaxed underwriting in a captive market is as good as or better than national insurance funded through taxation – only that it does not alter the moral or financial necessity of treating HIV patients.

Let us distinguish between the case where it is legally compulsory to insure oneself privately (a captive market) and the case where, because there is no welfare state, it is prudent to do so and many people are disposed to insure themselves privately (a quasi-captive market). Then quasi-captive markets for specialised insurance products can exist alongside an otherwise comprehensive state health insurance scheme. In the UK there is a quasi-captive market for life insurance in connection with mortgages, and for income support insurance for the self-employed. If the existence of captive markets strengthens the obligation of insurers to accept insurance applications from even the high-risk, including those at risk of contracting HIV disease, does the existence of quasi-captive markets give a reason for accepting applications for specialised insurance from the high-risk? If insurance is a means to the acquisition of something necessary for a decent rather than a luxurious standard of life, the answer can be 'Yes'. Permanent Health Insurance (PHI) policies and Critical Illness Insurance (CII) may be necessary to make up the income shortfall of self-employed people who are not high earners, and life insurance may be necessary to make up the shortfall in families if an income earner or *the* income earner dies.

In the UK, life insurance can be required for mortgages, which are in turn required for the purchase of accommodation. Ownership gives the best access to the most decent housing, and private rented housing is both expensive and scarce. The impact upon those who are HIV positive of being refused life insurance in connection with a mortgage is, therefore, severe.The difficulty of gaining good housing without access to mortgage facilities was recognised by the House of Commons Science and Technology Committee in 1995, in its report on the potential impact of genetic tests. It was acknowledged as 'an especially sensitive area'[2] by the Association of British Insurers in February 1997, when the ABI released a policy statement on life insurance and genetics. In this statement the ABI guaranteed that in applications to any of its members for life insurance in connection with a new mortgage application of up to £100,000 adverse genetic test results would be ignored for at least the next two years. This means that although account will still be taken of the family health history, those who actually test positive for some hereditary disorder (such as Huntington's disease) will not be refused life insurance on the basis of the test result alone. For the next two years at least, then, the industry should be able to maintain its much boasted record of providing life cover for 95 per cent of applications under standard terms. This generosity, however, was limited to genetic disorders. Despite the recognition which the House of Commons select committee and the ABI have given to the special problems of mortgages, no similar provisions have been made for those who are HIV positive.

Yet the same housing difficulties are faced by those who are HIV positive, or who are judged to be at risk of becoming HIV positive. If it is morally important for there to be wide access to this area – or other similar areas – of insurance, is it fair for this 'quasi-captive' market of near monopoly to be barred to anyone, or made difficult for anyone?

The insurance industry may be tempted to claim that even though the market for life insurance in connection with mortgages is large, it is not sufficiently large to outweigh the unprofitability of providing life cover for those who are HIV positive. This argument is considerably weakened by the existence of at least one American insurance company which *is* willing to insure those who are HIV positive. In April 1997, the US-based Guarantee Trust Life began offering life policies of between $25,000 and $250,000 to residents of Illinois who had tested HIV positive. In July of the same year it announced that it was willing to do the same in all states with the exception of New York, Florida and Alabama. It also announced that the minimum face value of such policies would be decreased to $10,000. In its July press release Guarantee Trust Life claimed that 'From an insurance perspective . . . many otherwise healthy HIV positive individuals are more appropriately treated as having a treatable chronic illness rather than a terminal disease.' This life cover comes at a price. An average policy for an HIV positive, non-smoking thirty-year-old male costs $300 a month.

Guarantee Trust Life operates in at least as fierce a market as companies do in the UK but has the additional disadvantage of operating in a society where rented accommodation is more plentiful and the attitude to home ownership is different from that in the UK, so that there is less of a captive market for life insurance in connection with mortgages. What is clear, though, is that it would not have extended cover to other states or decreased the minimum face value of policies if it was an inherently unprofitable market. It remains to be seen whether any UK companies will be prepared to follow this lead.

Other forms of insurance present problems similar to those just reviewed. Here are four examples. First, it is extremely difficult in the UK for the self-employed to gain access to state-funded income support even during periods of sickness, even though there has been an explosion in the number of small businesses and self-employment in the past fifteen years. Second, the serious financial impact of the incapacity of the main or sole child-care provider in families has been recognised by insurers, and policies worth from £1,560 to over £12,000 are available for those who have no formal income but work as so-called 'housepersons'. There is no state provision for funding the work that such persons do in a household should they fall ill or die. Third, the 1992–7 Conservative government made it more difficult for those who became unemployed (for whatever reason, including ill health) to secure their mortgage payments with state benefits. The market for insurance in connection with mortgage payments is now blossoming as some lenders insist that borrowers must take out such insurance as a condition of the loan. Finally, although there is state provision for families and individuals with no income at all, there is very little state help available to replace the income generated when one of the income earners dies. Many of those with children recognise the difficulties which would be faced by the surviving partner or the guardians in providing a home for their children on state benefits in the event of their death. Life insurance is, therefore, necessary for those who want to maintain a standard of living beyond the barest minimum for their children after their death.

In each of these cases, individuals refused insurance because they are HIV positive may thereby be seriously disadvantaged. The more seriously disadvantaged an individual is, the greater the obligation there is to meet his needs. But as the welfare state – in my view the best home for this obligation – continues to contract, and the market for private cover grows to meet the shortfall, it is arguable that the obligation of the industry to provide cover for those who are HIV positive should increase accordingly.

LIFESTYLE QUESTIONNAIRES AND
HIV TESTS

In the UK perhaps the most controversial aspect of HIV status and insurance has not been the obligation of the industry to provide insurance for everyone but the way in which the industry has gone about its legitimate business of assessing risk in relation to HIV infection. In 1993 the ABI recommended the following wording for the lifestyle questionnaire:

Have you ever
(a) been personally counselled or medically advised in connection with HIV (AIDS) or any sexually transmitted disease? (Please give dates and circumstances*)
or
(b) had an HIV (AIDS) test? (Please give dates, circumstances* and results)

*To enable the company to process this application as quickly as possible and to reduce the need for further investigations, please indicate whether counselling or test was for routine screening (e.g. for blood donation, antenatal, employment, occupational health) or other reasons.

This formulation attempted to take account of opposition, from such HIV pressure groups as the Terrance Higgins Trust, to insurers assuming that simply taking an HIV test was evidence of a high-risk applicant. The Terrance Higgins Trust pointed out – quite fairly – that HIV tests are taken for a variety of reasons including those described as routine in the 1993 formulation.

There is mounting evidence that insurance companies have changed their practice and are no longer charging people more if they have taken HIV tests, provided, of course, the results are negative. Undeniably, this is a change for the better. No one, least of all the insurance industry, would want to encourage a situation where the disadvantages of going for an HIV test outweighed the advantages – including the moral advantages of limiting the spread of this terrible virus. Even so, not all the industry is prepared to accept that low-risk groups of people may present themselves for testing. Spencer Leigh, formerly chief underwriter of Royal Insurance, has argued that only those who considered themselves at risk of being in contact with HIV would consider having an HIV test. This position fails to take into account that *everyone* engaging in penetrative sex with a new partner is at risk to some degree of contracting the virus. Surely, it is only legitimate for the industry to isolate those who are at greater risk than normal of so doing.

That some groups are at greater risk than others is actually reflected in the more recent standard lifestyle questionnaire, which actually lists the at-risk groupings (established by unspecified 'health authorities'). The lifestyle questionnaire draws attention to homosexual men, bisexual men, intravenous drug users (of non-prescribed drugs), haemophiliacs, those who have received blood or blood products outside the UK, and the sexual partners of all these groups.

The questionnaire still asks the following questions:

- Have you been tested or received medical advice or counselling or treatment in connection with AIDS or an AIDS-related condition? If yes, please give details, including names and addresses of doctors, and dates. (Routine testing for blood donation purposes may be ignored.)
- Have you ever been tested or received medical advice or treatment in condition with any sexually transmitted disease, including Hepatitis B? If yes, please give details, including names and addresses of doctors and dates.[3]

The questions remain substantially the same, and suggest that those who are extra-cautious are still in danger of being placed in a high at-risk group.[4] This penalises people for being responsible. Surely all of us who are sexually active are obliged, if we are responsible, to make sure that we are not HIV positive before having unprotected penetrative sex with new partners.

The current insurance industry questionnaire also requires people to disclose even the negative test results of tests taken for non-routine, highly sensitive and personal reasons unconnected with HIV high-risk groupings – such as in connection with infertility treatment, gamete donation or even rape and sexual assault. Without casting any doubt on the ability of the industry to maintain confidentiality within a secure information system, individuals may still be understandably reluctant to disclose a negative test result gained under these highly unusual circumstances. Yet, despite the fact that it would be unreasonable to suggest that any such individual is in a high-risk group, failure to disclose the test could result in problems claiming under the policy if the existence of the test became known.

There is some reason to think that lifestyle questionnaires should become more explicit about the sources of risk and not draw conclusions from previous negative tests or a history of sexually transmitted disease. The questionnaire procedure already depends on individuals being honest about their own sexual orientation and the known sexual orientation of their sexual partners. Since these highly personal disclosures are already required, it is only fair that the wrong conclusions should not be drawn from them. For instance, celibate homosexual men and homosexual men in permanent and long-term relationships are automatically considered to be in the high-risk groups, whilst there is no means of detecting promiscuous heterosexual individuals or people who sell sex, all of whom are probably at greater risk of contracting HIV disease. It is, of course, open to individuals to lie in response to questions designed to assess how promiscuous they are. But lying is a possibility for anyone. The real issue can be put by asking which questions are more likely to produce an accurate assessment of risk – and accordingly to be fairer – than the existing questions, and whether individuals who are prepared to be frank about their sexual orientation will not also be frank about sexual promiscuity. If heterosexuals are not being asked to disclose their sexuality or asked similarly searching questions, the claims of the homosexual community that it is being targeted unfairly gain credence.

HIV TESTS AS A PREREQUISITE OF INSURANCE

In order to obtain some forms of life insurance, individuals are asked to submit a negative HIV test result. Requests for such results are usually triggered when the life cover applied for is greater than £150,000 (in the case of single men) or £250,000 (in the case of married men or single women).[5] When smaller life policies are being applied for, clients will be asked for permission for the company to gain information from their GP-held medical records. General practitioners are then specifically asked to identify any health problems that may constitute a bad risk for life insurance, and some companies still ask GPs to comment on HIV risk, despite the British Medical Association's recommendation that GPs should always say that they never answer such questions. It is very difficult for GPs to deny knowledge of a positive HIV test. Some are even prepared to disclose negative test results, which has prompted many individuals to seek tests anonymously from walk-in clinics specialising in sexual transmitted diseases.

To its credit, the insurance industry has for some time now not only borne the costs of the tests themselves but also the cost of pre- and post-test counselling. The purpose of pre-test counselling is to remind individuals of the cost of having a positive test result, which goes beyond the immediate effect of being turned down for insurance. HIV disease and AIDS can result in stigma, ostracism and loss of family and friends. Pre-test counselling serves as a reminder to individuals that it may be beneficial to remain in ignorance.

Although there are practical benefits in not knowing that one is HIV positive, it is far from clear that individuals have a general right to remain in ignorance, even when others are not placed at an unfair risk as a result. Unfair risk in this context is usually associated with the risk of being infected by the virus. But in relation to insurance unfair risk lies elsewhere – in the scope insurance applicants have to underrepresent the risks they bring to the insurance pool. For this reason, some representatives of the industry have defended routine HIV testing on the grounds that those who have nothing to hide have nothing to fear – a formulation which itself does nothing to promote the image of sufferers from HIV disease or AIDS.

Current practice in the UK takes account of the background risk of infection within certain risk categories and depends upon the utmost good faith of the policyholders. The burden is on them to disclose factors relevant to risk, and if it turns out they have failed to do so the policy can be voided. Protection against large losses – which is to the benefit of all premium payers – is ensured by requiring a negative test for policies with a large face value. The freedom of individuals to remain in ignorance and still obtain insurance is protected because no test is required for smaller policies. The industry retains the right to investigate claims and refuse to pay out in the case of fraud, and to limit liability by limiting the face value of policies where no test is required. There is much to recommend current practice over either the extension of HIV tests to all life policies or the refusal to allow testing as a prerequisite of any policies.

HIV TESTS AND CLAIMS SETTLEMENT

As we have seen, current practice is based on utmost good faith and the entitlement of the industry to investigate all claims and refuse to pay out where claims are made fraudulently. But, it has been argued[6] the industry has different obligations when investigating deaths from HIV, particularly where the death was covered by a policy which required an HIV test. The financial and emotional effects of an investigation into a claim can be very great. Not only may the survivors of the policyholder be impoverished whilst waiting for a pay-out which they could legitimately expect to receive promptly, but where the death is AIDS-related they may also have to suffer insinuations about the sexuality and fidelity of partners or parents, not to mention worries about their own health and ostracism or prejudice from third parties drawn into the investigation of the claim. This level of distress is much greater than that generated by investigations concerning a non-HIV-related life claim, or burglary, etc. It would, therefore, undoubtedly be evidence of good practice for companies to put in place an infrastructure which encourages any investigations of AIDS-related deaths to be sensitive as well as impartial – if there *has* to be an investigation.

However sensitive a system of investigation may be, there is an additional question about whether it is fair to subject individuals to such a level of distress whilst simultaneously actively seeking every precaution at the underwriting stage. For this reason, there is a strong moral argument for the insurance industry to instigate a no-fuss settlement regime when a policy was issued only after a negative HIV test result was received. Utmost good faith is a two-way street which should offer protection to consumers as well as providers of insurance.

PERMANENT HEALTH INSURANCE AND CRITICAL ILLNESS INSURANCE

According to the report on health insurance by the Office of Fair Trading,[7] of the forty-six companies offering Permanent Health Insurance (PHI) examined, seventeen exclude disability caused by HIV infection, fifteen have policies which lapse once HIV infection is established and eleven specify that no benefit will be paid once it has been established.[8] Critical Illness (CII) policies, on the other hand, may cover HIV infection provided that the insured is a medical professional and the infection was contracted in the course of his or her work, or provided that it was contracted through a blood transfusion. Other emergency service (police, fire, ambulance) personnel may also be able to take out cover which includes HIV infection during the course of professional activities. There are several issues particularly related to HIV which these polices present for those professionals seeking cover.

1. Workers making a claim are going to have to prove that their infection has occurred during their professional activities. The standard way of doing this is for workers who fear that they have come in contact with the virus to arrange to have an immediate HIV test, and a further test six to eight weeks later. If the first test is negative and the second positive, it is not unreasonable to assume – all things being equal – that the infection occurred as a result of the reported event. However, this will inevitably lead to an increased number of HIV tests for the individual, each of which – even if negative – will have to be declared on future applications for life cover. There is a danger that the cautious policyholder, anxious to fulfil the requirements of one insurance company, will begin to look like a high-risk client to another company. It would be unjust if, as a result of taking out one policy, an individual's freedom to change other policies was curtailed. It would be particularly regrettable if applications were being made as a result of a change of housing and therefore mortgage arrangements.

2. Workers who are infected with HIV during the course of their professional activities are entitled to compensation from their employer – provided that safety regulations have been followed. Such compensation would usually take the form of a lump sum for the employee to spend on immediate needs or invest to yield an income. Such a pay-out may disadvantage someone with CII. Not all companies disregard unearned income (including interest payments) when working out how much a claimant is entitled to. This effectively means that they are refusing to cover double liability. If the employee's employer has to pay out compensation for HIV infection, the insurance company will be prepared only to top up the claimant's income to the insured level, instead of paying out on the whole sum insured and thereby leaving the employee with the benefit of both the income insurance and the compensation for HIV infection. Refusing double liability is already considered a dubious practice. The industry argues that it is wrong for an individual to benefit more than once from the same incident. However, individuals who benefit more than once benefit because they have paid more than once, and it is arguable that, having paid, they are entitled to claim. In addition to effectively refusing double liability, most insurance companies also include state benefits

when determining how much they are prepared to pay out to the unfortunate claimant. This means that many policyholders are over-insured, because they have been paying premiums on the basis of their total earnings rather than their earnings minus state or other benefits. It is not always clear from marketing information, however, that what the insurance companies are offering is to top up income when state benefits and legally required compensation have been taken into account. According to the Office of Fair Trading, the issue of how much a policyholder is entitled to is only really addressed when they come to claim. It would, therefore, be good practice for companies to inform individuals in advance of taking out a policy how much insurance – if any – they are actually likely to need. This is particularly important in the case of HIV because it is one of the few critical conditions that one can actually acquire during the course of one's work (the remainder include disabilities rather than illness), and undoubtedly some of the health care workers attracted to CII are attracted because of the HIV cover available to them.

3. The definition of 'total disability' varies from one company to another. Some companies reject claims if the claimant is able to engage in other activities for reward or profit. This is of particular importance to health care workers such as doctors, who may be required by their professional body to cease practising if they become HIV infected. Yet most would still be considered fit for other work, particularly in the short term. However, such work is not likely to be at the same rate of pay as the previous employment. Even if the individual was able to find other work within his or her profession it would inevitably be at a more junior level. Individuals who have been paying premiums to guarantee their level of income may find that their claim is rejected on the basis that they are still able to work. Even if the individual continued to pay premiums in the hope that this would eventually pay off when they were totally unable to work, the claim would then be settled only in relation to the existing income. Moreover, some companies require policy-holders to inform them of a change of occupation and will not necessarily continue cover in changed circumstances. This would provide an insurance company with the opportunity to discontinue a policy once the HIV infection was disclosed as a result of a failed claim.

4. Both PHI and CII types of policies are aggressively under-written and rejected at the application stage. Between 10 and 15 per cent of applications for CII,[9] and up to 25 per cent of those for PHI, are rejected; others have cover restricted for medical

reasons.[10] PHI premiums are loaded according to occupation and sex. (Women can expect to pay 25–65 per cent more than men.)[11] In the case of CII cover, premiums are also loaded according to age and sex[12] as well as by the range of cover offered (for instance, a greater or lesser number of conditions covered). Despite this rigour at the application stage, about 20 per cent of claims for CII cover are rejected[13] and 25 per cent of claims for PHI.[14] This is in part due to misunderstandings about what is covered, and to a moratorium approach to underwriting which is also criticised in the report.[15]

The moratorium approach does not require any physical examination or GP's report to be submitted. Insurance is given on the understanding that there is a moratorium on pre-existing conditions. This is an invitation to problems with claim settlement. Although it is reasonable for the insurance company to expect people to remember that they consulted a doctor in the last two years, it is less reasonable for patients to predict that a consultation over some minor problem (like a sore throat) was actually the first presentation of something much more sinister. Those who are at low risk of becoming HIV infected, or have no knowledge of the very early symptoms, may be disadvantaged in this way, as it may be some time before HIV is considered a possible explanation for continuing ill health. It is, therefore, good practice for insurance companies to insist on medical examinations or a report from a client's GP so that any pre-existing conditions are identified and excluded or underwritten.

The rate at which claims are rejected is worrisome in the case of HIV because it is actually very difficult to prove beyond doubt that the infection occurred at work. Some claimants – particularly homosexual men – are especially vulnerable in this respect. Yet, when there is a high rate of rejection and underwriting according to occupation with the additional protection of utmost good faith, it would be more ethical to establish no-fuss settlements particularly in relation to HIV by the few companies willing to cover this infection.

The insurance industry is under no obligation to provide a superior service to health care and other workers with an occupational risk of becoming HIV infected. It is not unreasonable, however, to expect individual companies to highlight the particular problems which may be generated when such workers take out these policies. The Office of Fair Trading has already recommended that greater care needs to be taken when helping individuals to calculate the amount of cover they need. This obligation is even greater if the policies are deliberately aimed at workers who may become HIV infected during the course of their employment.

NOTES

Some lines of thought in this chapter have their origins in a paper written with Tom Sorell in 1993: see 'HIV and insurance', in R. Bennett and C. Erin (eds), *Whispered Everywhere: HIV, Screening, Testing and Confidentiality*, Oxford, Oxford University Press (forthcoming). This chapter updates some of the information upon which those lines of thought were based. Tom Sorell also made valuable comments on the first draft of this chapter. Helpful information about companies offering Permanent Health Insurance and Critical Illness Insurance was provided by Howell Shone Insurance Brokers, Stoke on Trent. Guarantee Trust Life kindly faxed me their press releases of April and July 1997.

1 The fact that the NHS provides medical care does not mean that HIV/AIDS patients will be treated without stigma, or receive treatment tailored to all their needs. That *something* is provided no matter what does not mean that what is provided is beyond criticism.
2 Association of British Insurers, *Life Insurance and Genetics: A Policy Statement*, London, February 1997, p. 1.
3 This is the formulation of questions asked by Abbey National Life, and was kindly supplied by Ivan Massow Associates, London.
4 This was one of the points made in the paper by T. Sorell and H. Draper in Bennett and Erin, *Whispered Everywhere*, cited in note 1.
5 *AIDS Bulletin* No. 5 1991 (London: Institute of Actuaries), p. 20.
6 See Sorell and Draper, cited in note 1.
7 Office of Fair Trading, *Health Insurance*, London, HMSO, July 1996.
8 Ibid., p. 59.
9 Ibid., p. 75.
10 Ibid., p. 54.
11 Ibid., p. 54.
12 Ibid., p. 74.
13 Ibid., p. 75.
14 Ibid., p. 55.
15 The moratorium approach to private medical insurance is criticised in ibid., pp. 33–4, and its use in PHI is criticised on p. 66.

Part II

PUBLIC OR PRIVATE
PROVISION?

6

DISABILITY AND INSURANCE

Paul Fenn and Stephen Diacon

People with disabilities constitute as varied and diverse a population as any group of the able-bodied. Disability is found among people of all ages and all social backgrounds, and the extent of disability ranges from the relatively minor to conditions that involve dependence on others for meeting the most basic of daily needs. Recent estimates suggest that almost eleven per cent (that is, 3.8 million) of the working-age population in private households in Britain have a work-limiting long-term health problem or disability (Sly and Duxbury, 1995) and there may be as many as 6.5 million disabled people in the UK altogether (Armitage, 1997).

Official statistics on the prevalence of disability can be misleading because they tend to focus on those people who claim some type of disability benefit under the UK social security system. There are thought to be 1.5 million adults of working age in Britain claiming one or more of the four main disability benefits (Invalidity Benefit, Disability Living Allowance, Income Support with a disability premium or higher pension premium, and Severe Disablement Allowance), and the total spending on disability constitutes almost a quarter of the social security budget (Rowlingson and Berthoud, 1996). The vast majority of those receiving benefit were deemed to be incapable of work, and indeed Sly and Duxbury (1995) estimate that almost 70 per cent of the people with disabilities or work-limiting health problems were not in work.

To define disability is both a complex and a contentious task. The Disability Discrimination Act 1995, which came into force on 2 December 1996, defines a person as disabled if he 'has a physical or mental impairment which has a substantial and long-term adverse effect on his ability to carry out normal day-to-day activities'. In

116

other words, someone is disabled if they are unable, by virtue of some mental or physical impairment, to perform certain basic tasks such as walking, seeing, hearing, etc. In this so-called 'medical model', disabled people are the victims of an individual personal tragedy (of disease, heredity or accident), and such impairments are the direct cause of any resulting social or economic disadvantage or discrimination (Barnes, 1991). The two main definitions of disability used in the insurance industry are along the same lines: disability is generally defined either as the inability to follow any gainful occupation for which the person is suited, or the inability to perform the major duties of the person's own regular occupation (for example, see Diacon and Carter, 1992).

An alternative view of disability, known as the 'social model', is that the disabled are unable to 'carry out normal day-to-day activities' because society fails to accommodate people with different levels and types of ability. Thus it is the lack of flexibility and adaptability of current economic and social institutions (such as transport, housing, insurance, etc.) that prevents disabled people from living normal lives rather than their physical or mental impairments *per se*. In contrast to the medical model, the causes of disadvantage and discrimination arise from the failure of other people, systems and institutions to cope with the full diversity of human needs.

Rowlingson and Berthoud (1996) note that the social model of disability is currently the minority, rather than the mainstream, view. However, this picture is likely to change as a result of the development of genetic screening technology, which can in principle detect whether individuals are at increased risk from a disease or condition which is likely to disable them *in the future*. People who have a latent disability may well find that they are disadvantaged, not because of any current mental or physical impairment (which by definition is not readily observable), but because of the unwillingness of others to accord them the goods, services and facilities they need now as a result of their increased risk of disability in the future. To some extent, people with latent disabilities may thus experience discrimination in the same way as those who already suffer a disabling condition or impairment – thus creating what has been termed a 'genetic underclass' (Cookson, 1997). Clearly the main problems will arise in the transaction of long-term contracts (such as house purchase, bank loans, adoption, military service) where the ability of people with latent disabilities to perform in the future (for example, to continue to make loan repayments) is in doubt. The most obvious illustration of such problems arises when considering the operation of insurance and pension contracts.

INSURANCE AND DISABILITY

For many disabled people, insurance represents the means by which they are able to live a fulfilled life, free from financial insecurity, with the help of payments from a policy which provided benefits from the onset of their disability. But insurance is not available to all the disabled – those disabled from birth, for example – and those who are eligible do not always obtain insurance easily. A survey of disabled people, undertaken before the Disability Discrimination Act 1995 came into force, reported that 60 per cent of respondents had trouble obtaining health insurance, 58 per cent had difficulty finding life insurance and even 45 per cent experienced problems with motor insurance (Armitage, 1997). In fact, there are at least two ways in which people who are already disabled are affected by the behaviour of insurers:

- For those who have a pre-existing condition, cover is often not available against the consequences of disability, such as through medical insurance, permanent health insurance, or critical illness cover.
- For those who are disabled and who wish to buy other insurance policies, such as life insurance, motor vehicle insurance, or household contents insurance, the insurer can refuse cover or load premiums in relation to the insured's disability (although the increased risk of early death may mean that annuity rates are reduced).

The flip side of the coin is that insurers will often afford better treatment to those people who can demonstrate that they are healthier than average. These 'preferred lives' may be charged less for cover under life insurance, private medical insurance, etc., but may pay more for annuities. Clearly, the differential treatment of insureds on grounds of their disability raises ethical questions. In the UK these ethical questions have recently been engaged by the Disability Discrimination Act 1995.

The possibility that someone may have a latent disability (in the form of an increased risk of future disability) may also cause insurers to deny cover or increase premiums if the risk to the insurer is higher during the period of the policy. For many years, insurers have attempted to predict the existence of latent disability by examining the insured's health record and family history. Insurers have traditionally asked questions about the causes of death of the insured's parents and nearest blood relatives, and have tried to establish whether they had suffered from any hereditary illnesses. Nowadays the possibility of using the results from genetic tests (which may indicate a genetic susceptibility to disease) has emerged as a crucial issue in the insurer's underwriting decisions. Some commentators reject the value of genetic tests, so that the marketing manager of one UK life insurer was able to assert that 'family history already tells insurers all they need to know to underwrite successfully and it will be ten years before genetic tests become sophisticated enough to have a big impact on risk assessment' (Adams, 1997). Others are less sanguine, and a recent editorial notes that, although genetic testing currently reveals little more about health prospects than family history, actuaries expect that in ten to twenty years' time full-scale tests will be able to predict a threefold difference in mortality between people with good and bad genes (*Financial Times*, 19 February 1997).

THE DISABILITY DISCRIMINATION ACT 1995

Prior to the introduction of the Disability Discrimination Act 1995 (hereafter 'the Act' or 'DDA 1995') the insurance market's attitude towards people with disabilities appeared to be one of prejudice and ignorance, and this in turn generated much antagonism and ill feeling. The standard insurance terms for people with existing or latent disabilities, including 'impaired' and 'substandard' lives, are a public relations disaster in themselves. Research undertaken by bodies such as the Royal Association for Disability and Rehabilitation frequently indicated that insurers commonly denied cover and/or charged high prices to people with disabilities – often without providing any explanation or justification. Furthermore, insurers were often accused of not understanding the nature of disability, and of being unduly intrusive in their information requirements before cover could be offered. Finally, disabled people often experienced practical difficulties in the process of purchasing their insurance policies (for example, in finding out which insurer to approach, filling in the application form, understanding the terms and conditions, and in obtaining advice) and in making a claim.

The Act was introduced somewhat hurriedly only six months after the publication of a consultative document. Gooding (1996) notes that it should therefore be regarded as a framework which can be progressively extended, restricted or clarified through regulations subsequent to its enactment. While the consultative document originally proposed that insurance should be excluded from the section of the Act which deals with the right of access to goods and services, the statute as enacted did not make this exclusion. Hence insurance is covered by the provisions of Part III of the Act, which prohibits discrimination against disabled people in the provision of services, goods or facilities. Section 20 (1) explains that service providers discriminate against a disabled person if, for a reason which relates to the disabled person's disability, he is treated less favourably than others to whom that reason does not apply – in a way which cannot be justified under the provisions of the Act.

Sections 20 (3) and (4) say that differential treatment is justified if, in the opinion of the service provider (where it is reasonable to hold such an opinion):

> the difference in the terms on which the service is provided to the disabled person and those on which it is provided to other members of the public reflects the greater cost to the provider of services in providing the service to the disabled person.
>
> (20 (4) (e))

In addition, in relation to the refusal to provide services to disabled people, a further justification is:

> because the provider of services would otherwise be unable to provide the service to members of the public.
>
> (20 (4) (c))

Clearly, these justifications are sufficiently broad that some clarification is needed with respect to insurance practice. The supplementary regulations clarifying the interpretation of justifiable treatment in the provision of insurance came into force on 2 December 1996 (SI 1996 1836). Regulation 2 specifies that insurers may be justified in treating a disabled person less favourably if the treatment is

> based upon information (for example, actuarial or statistical data or a medical report) which is relevant to the

assessment of the risk to be insured and is from a source on which it is reasonable to rely, and reasonable having regard to the information relied upon and any other relevant factors.

This requirement relates to new policies sold after 2 December 1996. Regulations 3 and 4 of the statutory instrument relate to the transitional arrangements which must apply to existing policies and cover notes.

Although it is still too early to tell precisely how the provisions of the Act will affect the UK insurance industry, it is possible to draw one or two tentative conclusions. In the first place, insurers must ensure that they comply with the Act both in terms of the fundamentals of underwriting, cover and premium rating and also in terms of access to their premises and other facilities. Second, insurers will have to take care to ensure that any differential treatment can be fully justified with statistical or other relevant evidence. Gooding (1996) notes that the supplementary regulations which justify less favourable treatment were not intended to provide insurers with a convenient 'opt out' from the main provisions of the Act.

Finally, it is clear that the supplementary regulations present insurers with a difficult decision, since they must either treat disabled and able-bodied people in the same way or seek to justify any less favourable treatment. Prior to the Act becoming law, insurers who differentiated their premiums could in principle do so without recourse to especially detailed actuarial calculations. Now those insurers have two choices: they can stop differentiating their premiums; or they can invest in 'reasonable' actuarial or statistical analysis, which may therefore result in changes to the previous premium structure. It follows that there is a possibility that some disabled people – those who are newly rated at a higher premium as a consequence of the Act – will actually lose out as a result of the legislation. By contrast, those disabled people who are newly rated alongside the able-bodied (as a result of their insurer switching to a pooled premium) will gain as a consequence of the Act. Clearly, the extent to which insurers respond to the requirements of the Act, and the effect on the welfare of insureds, will depend on the availability of information in relation to the risks associated with disability. Acquiring this information will obviously involve insurers in additional costs in compiling the necessary databases, and they will always be subject to the criticism that their analyses are not thorough enough to distinguish adequately the many different types and degrees of disability. As Armitage (1996) puts it:

> the number, range and severity of disabilities is so vast, and their effects dependent on such varying factors, that any underwriter is going to find it difficult to compile statistics that would stand up in court.

INSURANCE, EFFICIENCY AND EQUITY

Clearly, the differential treatment of insureds on grounds of their (current or latent) disability raises ethical questions. We now consider in general terms the normative arguments for and against the differential treatment of some individuals relative to others by insurers. We consider these arguments in relation to the concepts of efficiency and equity.

Efficiency

Imagine a society in which there are only two types of individual, A and B, identical apart from the fact that A has a disability (which may be current or latent) which is associated with a one-in-four chance of being incapacitated for work. Consequently B's lifetime income flow is certain, whereas A's is uncertain. Would B agree to share some of A's risk by undertaking to pay him a sum of money in the event that he develops the incapacity? The answer to this question of course depends on what motivates individual B: is he concerned only with his own well-being or is he concerned also for the well-being of A? Leaving the issue of altruism on one side for the moment, it may well be in both individuals' mutual self-interest to negotiate an arrangement whereby some of the risk of incapacity is transferred to B in exchange for a payment from A. This concept of mutually beneficial exchange leads to a normative principle closely linked with utilitarianism: society as a whole will be better off if mutually beneficial gains from trade are exploited – this is the concept of (Pareto) efficiency. A wider definition of efficiency applies if the sharing of risk takes place *without* a payment from A: if A's gain in well-being from the reduction of risk outweighs B's loss from the increase in risk, we could argue that society as a whole is better off – this is the concept of 'Hicks–Kaldor' efficiency.

It is tempting to read into this example the structure of an insurance contract, so that B is an insurer offering contingent benefits to A in exchange for a consideration in the form of a premium. However, in a simple two-person society it is likely that both individuals will have a distaste for risk, and that will reduce considerably the scope for trade. The role of insurance becomes clearer if we envisage a society with a large number of individuals like A. If B decides to offer an insurance contract as above which is purchased by many A-type individuals, then in any one year B will have an income from the premiums, and will incur liabilities only to those As who are incapable of work in that particular year. The losses of the few, then, are, in effect, paid by the many. As a result, the lifetime income stream of B could be very stable from year to year if the risks to the As are independent of each other. This is known as the *law of large numbers* and is a fundamental principle of insurance. As a result of the pooling of benefits from large numbers, the scope for efficient trade between insurers and individuals facing risk is considerably enhanced.

Consider next the possibility that individuals C possess a disability which is associated with a one-in-two chance of being incapacitated for work. Assuming that the insurer has a means of finding out the difference between individuals A and C, it has two options. It could work out what premium would be needed to charge for cover to both A and C in order that its income and liabilities should balance in any given year – this is a *pooling contract* involving a degree of cross-subsidisation from the low-risk As to the high-risk Cs. While this arrangement could be seen as equitable, in that both A and C pay the same premium, we will argue that it is inefficient. Alternatively the insurer could work out what distinct premiums could be charged to As and Cs separately so that the income from each risk type as a group balances the liabilities from each risk type as a group: that is, the insurer would avoid cross-subsidisation between risk types by using *separating contracts* (or premium discrimination). If the insurer is indeed able to differentiate between risk types at negligible cost, it is surely efficient for it to do so: otherwise there will be a gap between the expected cost of the contract to the insurer in terms of claims and the expected value of the contract to the insured, and this would imply some further potential gains from trade. As far as efficiency is concerned, it can be shown that an insurance market in which everyone pays a per unit premium equal to his or her expected loss is one in which all potential gains from trade have been exhausted.

Many of the ethical issues in relation to disability and insurance stem from this distinction between pooling and separating contracts. To begin with, there is often a confusion between the insurer's role in pooling risks *over time* (that is, the law of large numbers), and the desirability of pooling *across individuals* who face different risks. It is often not fully understood that an insurer is quite capable in principle of charging a separate and distinct premium to every individual while still carrying out the pooling function associated with insurance.

Equity

What, then, are the ethical difficulties with separating contracts? Why should insurers be challenged on moral grounds when differentiating between insureds on grounds of actual disability, or a known propensity to become disabled? To begin with, it could be argued that disability is a fundamental characteristic of individuals, like their sex and race, over which they have no control, and it is therefore somehow 'unfair' or inequitable for the disabled to be treated any differently from people without disabilities (see Sen, 1985, for a discussion of the relationship between justice and the distribution of basic capabilities of people). Related to this is the argument that differentiation can be used in some contexts as a vehicle for uninformed prejudice. For example Black and Skipper (1994) report the results of a 1990 public attitude survey, undertaken on behalf of the American Council of Life Insurance, which asked whether it was fair to charge premiums which depended on the insured's social, economic and medical characteristics. Although the majority of respondents agreed that it was fair to vary premiums according to characteristics over which the insured had some control (such as smoking behaviour, hobbies, occupation, etc.) there was very little support for differentiation according to factors over which the insured had little control (such as a genetic predisposition to cancer). Equity in this sense is concerned with the protection of fundamental rights to non-discriminatory treatment.

Alternatively, it could be maintained that there is a societal preference for partial redistribution from those bearing low risks to those bearing high risks through no fault of their own – if egalitarian values are defined in terms of expected wealth (and this preference would be reinforced if there was an observed negative correlation between risk and wealth). For example, people who have been born with a particular disability such as cerebral palsy may have been unable to work for any length of time, and for that reason they may have relatively low wealth in conjunction with an uncertain future. If low-risk, high-wealth individuals cross-subsidise such individuals through pooling contracts, it might be seen as a fair outcome by many people. This is closer to the economist's usual use of the term 'equity', in the sense of distributive justice.

In either of these senses, it could be argued that discriminatory premiums in favour of the able-bodied are inequitable, even if they could be shown to be efficient. However, we now proceed by asking whether insurers are indeed acting as moral agents when differentiating between risk groups: that is, we consider in the next section whether insurers are forced into adopting particular premium structures in the light of competitive market pressures.

INSURANCE, INFORMATION AND COMPETITION

Full information and disclosure

Where insurers have full information about insureds (that is, where that information is publicly available at negligible cost), they are forced through competition to charge a premium which accurately reflects differences in risk – a practice variously known as risk classification or premium discrimination (for example, see Diacon, 1990, chapter 12). Any attempt by an insurer to cross-subsidise the high-risk individuals (by raising charges to the low-risk ones) will be frustrated by other insurers which will offer lower-priced contracts to the low-risk types.[1] Consequently the existence of a competitive market in insurance is one mechanism by which an efficient premium structure can be secured when information about risk types is publicly available. Of course, as discussed in the previous section, an efficient premium structure may be one which imposes severe loadings on those with serious disabilities, and there is an inevitable tension here between efficiency and equity.

To the extent that information about future risks or pre-existing conditions is held privately by individuals, insurers may be able to obtain this information at little cost if insureds are obliged to share it on agreeing a contract of insurance. Consequently, insurers require the completion of a detailed application (proposal) form before the insurance contract can be offered. The filling-in of the insurance proposal form is governed by the legal principle of utmost good faith (*uberrimae fidei*), which requires the proposer to disclose any information which may influence a prudent underwriter in determining the premium or deciding whether or not to take the risk (so-called 'material facts'). Further details on the law of disclosure can be found in Chapter 4 of Diacon and Carter (1992). The full legal situation is summed up in the judgement in the case of Rozanes *v.* Bowen (1928):

> As the underwriter knows nothing, and the man who comes to him to ask him to insure knows everything, it is the duty of the assured . . . to make a full disclosure without being asked of all the material circumstances. This is expressed by saying that it is a contract of utmost good faith.

In practice, the full rigours of the law of disclosure are ameliorated by the *Statements of Insurance Practice* adopted by members of the Association of British Insurers and Lloyd's underwriters in respect of individual proposers resident in the UK and insuring in their private capacity. The *Statements* require insurers to ask clear questions in the proposal form about those matters which are generally considered material, to draw attention to the consequences of failure to disclose all material facts, and to warn the proposer that if he is in any doubt about facts considered material he should disclose them. The *Statements* also require that all questions on the proposal forms should be answered to the best of the proposer's knowledge or belief.

The implication of the requirement to disclose all material facts is that the purchaser of insurance is required to answer all the insurer's questions truthfully ('according to the proposer's knowledge and belief') and reveal any other information which is likely to be important in the insurer's decision-making. For people with current or latent disabilities, the most crucial questions will be about their family medical history; however, the most controversial questions are likely to relate to the existence and results of any genetic tests which they have undertaken. The preceding discussion makes it clear that proposers have no option but to answer such questions in full. In February 1997 the Association of British Insurers published a policy statement (ABI, 1997) which recommended its members to require people wishing to take out new life insurance policies to report the results of any genetic tests which have already been undertaken (unless otherwise indicated). Although not all UK insurers may take this advice, the clear message from the ABI is that the insured's decision to take a genetic test, and the information so obtained, should be taken into account in determining the terms and conditions of any insurance contract. Those insurers which choose not to use test information in their underwriting decisions can expect to be placed at a competitive disadvantage, in comparison with those that do, as soon as the tests provide meaningful information which cannot be gleaned from family histories. For this reason it seems unlikely that the DDA 1995 will have had any significant effect on the use of disclosure by insurers. To the extent that the Act asks insurers to base underwriting practice on evidence, they will collect relevant facts from insureds at the proposal stage; however, there is every expectation that competitive pressures will force insurers to do all they can in this respect even in the absence of the Act. Whether they succeed in eliciting all private information from potential insureds is a moot point, and we now proceed to consider the implications if they fail.

Asymmetrical information and categorisation

In the absence of full disclosure (or where it is difficult to enforce) the insured individual may retain information which is denied to insurers. Since the insured individual has private information, he or she is able to use it to their advantage and to the detriment of the insurance pool: behaviour which is commonly known as adverse selection or anti-selection. A survey of some of the more significant results in the literature on adverse selection in insurance markets is available in Dionne and Doherty (1992).

Given asymmetrical information, an insurer's underwriting decisions can be improved by *categorising* individuals according to observable and reliable characteristics (such as age, medical history, gender) which are known to be statistically correlated with the (unobservable) risk. Some of these characteristics are so well accepted in the insurance community that they would certainly be classified as material facts. For example, in motor insurance the driver's age is known to be strongly negatively associated with the risk of an accident, so that all young drivers – no matter how safe they *actually* are – will be charged a higher premium. Since a motorist's predilection for dangerous sports such as sky diving or bungee jumping may be correlated with an unobservable reckless attitude to driving, insurers may want to take that into account as well; but it is unclear, in legal terms, when a mere statistical correlate becomes a material fact.

However, problems can emerge if underwriters are forced to become more detailed in their risk categorisation. In the first place, Gaulding (1995) notes that some anti-discrimination commentators do not regard mere statistical correlation as sufficient justification for categorisation: in order to avoid unfair discrimination, the insured's characteristics should also be causally connected with the risk measured, controllable by the insured, and not associated with historical or invidious discrimination. Second, detailed risk categorisation which identifies high-risk types more accurately (and then penalises them in terms of underwriting, cover and pricing) may restrict the availability of insurance in a way which many would regard as being contrary to the public good:

> destructive competition for the good risks is creating a new class of uninsurable risks. If we cannot offset the risks of chronic disablement, young drivers in fast cars or long-term industrial disease with a broad spectrum of more predictable risks, we may well find ourselves following the American example of government intervention in the insurance market.
>
> (Baird, 1997, quoting a leading UK insurance chief executive)

Notwithstanding these problems, it can be shown that costless categorisation of insureds is always efficient in the Hicks–Kaldor sense: that is, it is always possible for the gainers to compensate the losers (Crocker and Snow, 1986).[2] However, where categorisation involves a significant cost to the insurer, it is not always the case that such categorisation is efficient: whether it is or not clearly depends on the costs involved (Crocker and Snow, 1986). Consequently, even if the issue of equity is left aside, the social desirability of categorisation on the basis of disability, where the evidential requirements are potentially very high, is ambiguous at best. Moreover, competitive pressures may force insurers to categorise even when the winners from categorisation are unable in principle to compensate the losers (Crocker and Snow, 1986) Effectively, the market can fail to achieve efficiency because a given insurer's decision to categorise does not take into account the categorisation cost which is imposed on other insurers under the threat of cherry-picking.

On the face of it, this would seem to be an argument for the statutory prohibition of costly categorisation, such as discriminatory treatment of disabled people. However, the matter is not as straightforward as that. If categorisation is very costly, insurers will not categorise even in a competitive market, and that will be the efficient outcome. If categorisation costs very little, on the other hand, insurers will probably categorise, and that will also be efficient. It is the intermediate cost options which raise market failure problems, and it is not clear how to judge when such conditions are present. In fact what the DDA 1995 does is to prohibit *costless* categorisation on grounds of disability. Clearly, the equity objective of policymakers is dominant here, but it should be noted that this objective will be pursued at some loss of efficiency. Moreover, to the extent that the Act permits *costly* categorisation, through the use of actuarial or statistical analysis, we would argue that it may be tolerating some discrimination which is both inequitable and inefficient.

Asymmetrical information, signalling and screening

If the insurer is genuinely unable to distinguish between high-risk and low-risk individuals from the information provided in the proposal form, or is indeed prohibited by legislation from doing so, the next alternative may be to persuade individuals to reveal their risk status voluntarily by utilising either signalling or screening devices.

In the *signalling* case, low-risk individuals may take the initiative to indicate their status to the insurer so that they can be treated beneficially. Since high-risk individuals may also wish to represent themselves as low-risk, the signal will be believed only if it is sufficiently costly (since only low-risk individuals have an incentive to send costly signals). For example, in order to signal their above-average driving ability, disabled motorists could volunteer to take an advanced driving test which, if passed successfully, might induce the insurer to offer better terms.

In the *screening* case, the insurer may take the initiative to design contracts which will induce individuals to reveal their status. Rothschild and Stiglitz (1976) explain that, in some circumstances, it may be possible to obtain a stable equilibrium in a competitive insurance market by using separating price/quantity contracts as a screening device, so that high-risk and low-risk individuals 'self-select' the contract most suitable for themselves (in effect, low-risk individuals opt for policies which have low premiums and high deductibles). However, in other circumstances – particularly when the proportion of high-risk individuals in the community is small – Rothschild and Stiglitz show that it is not possible to obtain stability in insurance markets using separating price/quantity contracts. Other economists have sought to show that contracts with some degree of pooling, or cross-subsidisation, may emerge in a competitive equilibrium (Wilson, 1977; Miyazaki, 1977). Furthermore the whole concept of a price/quantity contract relies on the insurer's ability to monitor the amount of cover that the individual purchases from *other* insurers – something which can be very difficult to achieve in practice.[3]

Consequently, insurers who are deterred from adopting discriminatory premiums as a result of the DDA 1995 may instead adopt a screening strategy under pressure of competition.[4] Whether or not this is efficient will, as we have seen, depend on how costly it was to differentiate risk types prior to the Act. Whether or not it is equitable depends on how society trades off the welfare gains and losses which result. For example, some people may have been placed inappropriately into a high-risk group by insurers adopting crude categorisation prior to the Act, and that might be viewed as inequitable. However, if after the prohibition of such practices, insurers effectively screen out low-risk types by the use of price/quantity contracts, the same individual may find that he is induced to buy a contract which, while it has a lower premium, is nevertheless constrained in the amount of cover available (i.e. it has a high compulsory deductible). An example of this development would be if insurers who are deterred from loading PHI premiums on grounds of disability began to introduce wider premium differentials based on the benefits or deferred periods chosen by the insured. It is not evident who would be the gainers and losers under this scenario; what seems clear is that there would be some losers, and that some of those losers could be disabled individuals themselves, forced to pay higher premiums as a result of increased screening by insurers.

CONCLUSION

We have argued in this chapter that there are 'good' utilitarian reasons why insurers should be allowed to treat disabled and able-bodied people differently if they have relevant information about relative risk. Those reasons are based on efficiency arguments: effectively, scarce insurance capacity is best utilised by ensuring that its price reflects the cost to the insurer of taking on the extra risk. Moreover, the competitive nature of insurance markets may ensure that insurers have to set their premiums to reflect cost; otherwise they may go out of business. However, there are three important considerations which should qualify this position.

First, there could be principles of equity at issue which conflict with principles of efficiency, and which therefore result in pressure for either self-regulation or government legislation such as the Disability Discrimination Act 1995 in the UK. Then, provided that all insurers must comply with anti-discriminatory regulations, the competitive pressure to differentiate premiums could be withstood. However, it should be noted that insurance is increasingly sold across national boundaries, such that competitive pressures may remain a factor. Second, if the means by which insurers place people into different categories for insurance purposes involve non-negligible costs (such as through a medical examination), it has been shown (for example by Crocker and Snow, 1986) that competitive pressures could force insurers to categorise when it is *inefficient* to do so (the gainers could not compensate the losers from categorisation). Third, if insurers are unable to categorise people explicitly because of legislation such as the DDA 1995, they may turn under pressure of competition to the use of screening methods in order to differentiate between risk types implicitly through contracts with varying degrees of cover.

Taking these points together, what is the likely impact of the 1995 Act? Because it allows 'justifiable' discrimination, it is clearly feasible for insurers to continue to offer less favourable terms to disabled people. However, they must now do so only on the basis of 'reasonable' evidence. It is no longer possible to load premiums for those with a disability unless some medical, actuarial or statistical analysis has been undertaken. In effect, the Act ensures that differentiation can *only* take place provided that a cost has been incurred first. In the light of the Crocker and Snow arguments, such differentiation between disabled and able-bodied individuals may be both inefficient *and* inequitable. On this view, the outcome of the Act may simply be to force more insurers to incur actuarial costs which ensure continuing (and perhaps more extensive) discrimination against disabled people but which are not justifiable on efficiency grounds: the worst of both worlds! Of course, the extent to which that happens will, among other things, depend on the way in which the courts interpret and enforce the Act, and the way in which insurers respond to their judgements. Of particular importance is the kind of actuarial evidence which is considered 'reasonable' for the insurer to rely on. If the courts insist on a much higher standard of evidence than is currently the norm, insurers will probably simply stop charging differential premiums. If instead they reflect what is current practice amongst those insurers which use actuarial evidence, the Act may result in other insurers adopting this practice as a benchmark when assessing premiums. Either way, there may be a need for litigation before the full effects of the Act are known. Of course, if the Act does succeed in driving insurers away from explicit discrimination, one possible consequence is that we will observe a significant shift towards implicit discrimination in the form of screening behaviour. Disabled people may find that the Act in their name is something of a double-edged sword.

NOTES

1 Of course cross-subsidising pooling contracts may still be possible in insurance markets with full information, but only if insurers are prevented from offering better terms and conditions to low-risk individuals and low-risk insureds are prevented, or can be dissuaded, from buying their cover elsewhere (i.e. if the market is not perfectly competitive). The possible consequences are graphically illustrated by Finsinger et al. (1985), who describe how attempts to prevent premium discrimination in West German motor insurance markets in the 1970s and 1980s led to high prices and anti-competitive behaviour – a situation which persisted until free trade under the EU forced German motor insurers to price competitively.

2 An example of categorisation which is effectively costless would be the automatic loading of premiums for female insureds, or those aged under twenty-five.

3 Moreover it should be noted that there are other forms of screening mechanism available to insurers. In particular, if information can be shared between insurers, or if binding contracts can be written over more than one time period, it may be possible for insurers to adjust premiums over time in relation to observed claims experience (D'Arcy and Doherty, 1990). In principle, therefore, disabled people who are in fact low insurance risks will reveal themselves as such over time.

4 Because screening allows insureds to choose whichever contract they prefer, whether or not they have a disability, such behaviour is not contrary to the provisions of the Act.

REFERENCES

Adams C. (1997) Big Insurers Break Ranks over Genetic Test Results, *Financial Times*, 19 February, London.

Armitage J. (1997) Insurers Fear Hardening of Disability Rules, *Post Magazine*, 16 January, London.

Association of British Insurers (1997) *Life Insurance and Genetics: A Policy Statement*, ABI, London, February.

Baird R. (1997) The Great Unwashed, *Post Magazine*, 13 March, London.

Barnes C. (1991) *Disabled People in Britain and Discrimination*, London, Hurst.

Black K. and Skipper II. (1994) *Life Insurance*, twelfth edition, Englewood Cliffs, N.J., Prentice Hall.

Browne M. (1992) Evidence of Adverse Selection in the Individual Health Insurance Market, *Journal of Risk and Insurance* 59, 13–33.

Cookson C. (1997) Genetic Research 'Threatens Liberty', *Financial Times*, 19 February, London.

Crocker K. and Snow A. (1986) The Efficiency Effects of Categorical Discrimination in the Insurance Industry, *Journal of Political Economy* 94, 321–44.

D'Arcy S. and Doherty N. (1990) Adverse Selection, Private Information, and Lowballing in Insurance Markets, *Journal of Business* 63, 145–64.

Diacon S. R. ed. (1990) *A Guide to Insurance Management*, London, Macmillan Press.

Diacon S. R. and Carter R. L. (1992) *Success in Insurance*, third edition, London, John Murray.

Dionne G. and Doherty N. (1992) Adverse Selection in Insurance Markets: a Selective Survey, in G. Dionne (ed.) *Contributions to Insurance Economics*, Boston, Mass., Kluwer Academic Press.

Ellsberg D. (1961) Risk, Ambiguity and the Savage Axioms, *Quarterly Journal of Economics* 75, 643–69.

Finsinger J., Hammond E. and Tapp J. (1985) Insurance: Competition or Regulation?, Institute of Fiscal Studies, Report Series 19, London, IFS.

Gaulding J. (1995) Race, Sex and Genetic Discrimination in Insurance: What's Fair?, *Cornell Law Review* 80, 1646–94.

Gooding C. (1996) *Blackstone's Guide to the Disability Discrimination Act 1995*, London, Blackstone Press.

Kunreuther H., Meszaros J., Hogarth R. and Spranca M. (1995) Ambiguity and Underwriter Decision Processes, *Journal of Economic Behavior and Organization* 26, 337–52.

Miyazaki H. (1977) The Rat Race and Internal Labour Markets, *Bell Journal of Economics* 8, 394–418.

Rothschild M. and Stiglitz J. (1976) Equilibrium in Competitive Insurance Markets: An Essay on the Economics of Imperfect Information, *Quarterly Journal of Economics* 90, 629–50.

Rowlingson K. and Berthoud R. (1996) *Disability, Benefits and Employment*, Research Report 54, Department of Social Security, London, HMSO.

Sankey K. (1996) Life Threatening?, *Post Magazine*, 4 April, London.

133

Sen A. (1985) *Commodities and Capabilities*, Amsterdam, North Holland.
Sly F. and Duxbury R. (1995) Disability and the Labour Market: Findings from the Labour Force Survey, *Labour Market Trends*, December, London, CSO.
Smith B. and Stutzer M. (1990) Adverse Selection, Aggregate Uncertainty, and the Role for Mutual Insurance Contracts, *Journal of Business* 63, 493–510.
Wilson C. (1977) A Model of Insurance Markets with Incomplete Information, *Journal of Economic Theory* 16, 167–207.

7

ETHICAL ISSUES IN SOCIAL INSURANCE FOR HEALTH

Albert Weale

A politically aware observer at the end of the nineteenth century surveying the emerging democracies would have said that the principal political conflicts of the twentieth century would be over issues arising from the unequal ownership of the means of production. Indeed, right into the middle of the twentieth century, it was common for commentators from a variety of political perspectives to predict a trend towards the socialisation of the means of production. Although Schumpeter (1942) wrote in a somewhat wistful tone, he was not alone when he forecast the inevitable demise of capitalism.

Yet, from our vantage point, it is clear that many of the most salient current political choices are not about the socialisation of the means of production but about the socialisation of the means of *consumption* (Heidenheimer *et al.*, 1990, p. 218), and in this field the socialisation of health care consumption has played a prominent part. Indeed, there is now no developed liberal democracy, apart from the United States, which has not socialised the consumption of health care in such a way that the vast bulk of citizens now pool the financial risks of ill health in a scheme of collectively regulated or financed social insurance, even if it is not known by that name.

To say this, however, is no more than to note a historical fact; it is not to provide an intellectual rationale. Historical choices, even historical choices made by most societies, may be wrong or misguided. To say that the consumption of health care has been socialised is not to say that it should have been socialised, let alone to say that it should continue to be socialised in the future. To assert this latter proposition, we need both to formulate the basic principle of modern health care organisation and to examine the challenges to which it is prone.

This basic principle can be simply stated. It is that comprehensive, high-quality medical care should be available to all citizens on a test of professionally judged medical need and without financial barriers to access. There are a variety of organisational forms through which the principle may be implemented, including that of a tax-based public service as in the UK or the Nordic countries, tax-financed insurance as in Canada, or legally required compulsory social insurance as in Germany. In their different ways all three forms of organisation can be regarded as compatible with the principle of comprehensive, high-quality care available to all on a test of professionally judged medical need.

Yet, despite the widespread implementation of this principle, its plausibility has come under strain in recent years from the rising costs of health care. These costs have been increasing for a number of reasons, including improvements in medical techniques, changing age profiles of populations and rising expectations about the quality of care, all in the face of political concern about the proportion of national income that is devoted to health, and social expenditure more generally.

As a consequence of growing concern about health care rationing, fundamental questions are being raised about the basis of public health care provision, and in particular whether it is still possible for governments to make the commitment to their citizens of comprehensive, high-quality care. Since 'ought' implies 'can', these questions of feasibility also raise ethical issues. If comprehensive, high-quality care cannot be made available to all, is it still justifiable for governments to make the promises they do? Can we continue to talk without irony of there being an entitlement to health that takes the form of a right of citizenship? The purpose of this chapter is to explore these questions.

Since the challenge to the ethical basis of public provision comes from the claim that health care resources need to be rationed, we need to be clear what we mean by rationing. In its most acute form, rationing within a health care system may be defined as an implicit or explicit policy decision to withhold specific measures of treatment or care on the grounds that their economic costs are prohibitive, even though the measures in question are thought to yield some medical benefit (Weale, 1995, p. 831). As such, rationing can apply to measures intended to prolong life or improve its quality.

Rationing in this sense is a denial of treatment. However, as Rudolf Klein (Klein *et al.*, 1996, pp. 11–12) has suggested, rationing can take less serious, but still important, forms. These include: rationing by dilution, in which the resources devoted to each individual are spread thinly, for example shorter appointments with a general practitioner; rationing by delay, for example waiting lists for non-urgent surgery; and rationing by deflection, as when a health service problem is classified as a problem for the social services.

Why should the issue of rationing pose a problem about the basic principle of publicly assured health care? That principle is that comprehensive, high-quality medical care should be available to all citizens on a test of professionally judged medical need and without financial barriers to access. In denying needed care to certain people, or in diluting the quality of care that is provided, rationing casts doubt upon the implementation of this principle in practice. If care is denied to certain citizens, on the grounds that the costs of treatment are simply too great, the principle that citizens should have access to care on grounds of need is undermined. Similarly, if certain treatments are excluded from coverage in public systems, as is sometimes suggested, the comprehensive basis of the public service is attacked. Finally, if rationing by dilution is allowed to occur, the quality of the service is called into question.

One way of thinking about these issues is to consider whether we do not have something like what logicians would call an inconsistent triad of propositions, any two of which are compatible with each other, but all three of which are inconsistent taken together. Thus it can be argued that a system of health care can be comprehensive and freely available but not of high quality; or it can be high-quality and available to all but not comprehensive; or it can be comprehensive and of high quality but not available to all. Whichever way one takes of resolving the contradiction, the prospects for the traditional principle of public provision do not look good.

But are we faced with these stark choices? Does the existence of rationing pose such a severe test to the principles of socialised medicine? In seeking to answer this question, my strategy will be as follows. I shall first consider the institutional features of publicly assured health care that provide the context within which the rationing dilemma arises, before going on to the nature of the ethical problems that the rationing debate raises for the ethics of public provision. I shall then look at each of the proposed resolutions of the contradictions embodied in the claim of an inconsistent triad underlying the principle of modern health care systems. Finally,

I shall argue that the conflict of goals contained in modern systems of health care insurance is no more than we should expect, given an understanding of the logic of policy discourse itself. That political choice involves a compromise of competing ideals should hardly come as a surprise.

INSURANCE OR PUBLIC SERVICE?

Within all economically developed societies, the state assumes at least some responsibility for assuring medical care for its citizens. Some members of society may not have sufficient resources to insure themselves or, if they have sufficient money, they may suffer a form of myopia which means they allocate inadequate resources to cover their health care needs. One solution here is to blanket in these difficult cases by socialising insurance either through the tax system, as in Canada, or through a system of non-profit sickness funds based on compulsory membership, as in Germany. These two ways of socialising insurance are the most common ways of correcting for the distributional deficiencies of the health care market (White, 1995, p. 61).

Neither of these solutions entails the public ownership of medical care resources (in practice, hospitals and health centres). That further step is taken in some countries (primarily the UK and the Nordic countries). The rationale for such public ownership cannot simply be that of correcting for the distributional failures of the private insurance market, since that goal would be accomplished by the socialisation of insurance. Instead it has to be based upon a judgement about the benfits of being able to plan the allocation of resources, including personnel, in a more integrated way than is allowed for otherwise.

Although there is this formal distinction between the insurance rationale for the socialisation of health care finance and the public service rationale of the political ownership of health care facilities, in practice both approaches are committed to the basic principle of socialised medicine that I have set out. The difference between the two approaches, to be sure, raises important issues of adminis-trative theory and practice, but from the point of view of the basic entitlements to which each gives rise, they are functionally equi-valent. Consequently, in what follows, I shall treat both schemes of social insurance and schemes of public ownership of health care facilities on a par.

As it happens, the debate about rationing has been extremely vigorous in the UK, because of the highly political role that the public ownership of health care resources creates for health care decisions. Since, under public ownership of health care resources, the amount devoted to health spending is a political decision, it is not surprising that the UK debate has been particularly vigorous. However, the debate has also been carried on in social insurance systems like that of the Netherlands, in particular in the deliberations of the Dekker Commission. So, although there are good reasons for thinking that the highly centralised system of health care management in the UK will intensify debate, the broad spread of interest in the issue of rationing across the world suggests that the issue is essentially one about the basic principle of modern health care systems.

That being the case, we now need to consider what may be involved in dealing with the conflict of principles that the rationing issue throws up. I have suggested that the principle of comprehensive, high-quality and universally available care may be regarded as an inconsistent triad. The usual way in which to deal with an inconsistent triad is to drop one of the elements. Which, if any, of the comprehensiveness, quality and availability tests should we drop?

SHOULD PUBLIC SCHEMES DROP THE PRINCIPLE OF AVAILABILITY?

It might seem that considering whether to drop the principle of availability was such an obvious breach with the underlying rationale of publicly assured health care that there was no need to consider it. However, it is worth looking at in some detail as a way of exploring the logic of the dilemma we face, if we seek to make the basis of provision less inclusive.

This option is, of course, the one offered by private insurance, and other chapters in this book touch upon some of the ethical dilemmas implicit in the provision of private health insurance. However, putting the issues briefly, the objection to relying upon private health insurance as the fundamental basis of health provision, as distinct from an element in a broader strategy, is both distributional and efficiency-based.

The distributional argument is that those excluded from coverage on grounds of poverty or a pre-existing condition that makes private insurance unaffordable do not enjoy the conditions of equal citizenship that a democratic society should promote. This is not to say that there is no place for user charges, either to raise revenue or to signal to health care consumers the costs that are being borne, but any such measures ought to be constrained by the principle that no charges ought to make access to health care unaffordable for even the poorest citizen.

It may be argued that there was too strong a notion of social solidarity implicit in this argument. There is no reason to assume that the concept of citizenship, resting as it does on the idea of political equality, need imply the degree of social solidarity that is implicit in socialised forms of health care. From one point of view, the distinction between the conditions of citizenship and the social solidarity associated with the collectivised consumption of health care is valid. 'One person, one vote' does not imply the right to a hospital bed in the event of need. On the other hand, it may equally be argued that there is a rather arid formalism in granting equal political citizenship to members of a society but not caring about the extent to which their health care needs are met. Equal individual political worth does not imply equal access to health care, but the notion of individual worth that would find lack of access for some to health care permissible does not seem self-evident, to say the least.

In any case, the pure distributional argument can be supplemented with the efficiency argument. Medical schemes based on private insurance are subject to well known problems of cost control arising from asymmetrical information and the barriers to entry into the medical professions created in order to control the quality of care. Together these conditions mean that clinicians necessarily have considerable autonomy of behaviour and that consumers are often likely to make the wrong purchases. Indeed, the existence of professional autonomy means that even knowledgeable consumers like insurance companies that take on the burden of purchasing health care for individuals are likely to make the wrong purchases, since they are not in a position to monitor some of the crucial practices of health care professionals. In particular, the suitability of particular diagnostic tests or clinical interventions is difficult to monitor, and may lead to over-purchase or inflated billing (Reinhardt, 1987).

Given this asymmetry of information, the medical care market is unlikely to achieve an efficient allocation of resources. The problem is compounded by the existence of spill-over effects, particularly in relation to infectious diseases. Vaccinations, housing improvements and clean water are all likely to be undersupplied in a market, given that the benefits are generally available as a pure public good but the cost of provision falls on individuals. In these circumstances few will have an incentive to make a contribution to the provision of the public good sufficient to generate an optimal supply.

The twin expectation is, therefore, that a purely private market in health care will typically oversupply expensive high-tech medicine and undersupply public health care, including sanitation, housing improvements and vaccinations. In other words, market failure in health care means that we arrive at a situation not unlike the suppression of markets in most commodities in communist societies, where some goods were oversupplied and others undersupplied.

It is possible to imagine solutions to these problems arising within the insurance market itself. Indeed, such solutions have been put into practice, for example preferred-provider plans under which long-term contracts are established between insurers and providers according to guaranteed cost-schedules for patients falling into certain categories. However, although these arrangements address some of the problems, they do not address them all.

Universal availability is therefore not such an easy principle to drop in favour of a pure market approach. Hence we have to consider whether another element of the inconsistent triad should be jettisoned.

SHOULD PUBLIC SCHEMES DROP THE COMMITMENT TO COMPREHENSIVENESS?

Faced with the need to ration health care resources, one response has been a search for the elimination of inappropriate or ineffective treatments. If only, the proponents of this strategy say, we could get rid of expenditure on the things that public health systems should not be doing at all, we could then leave room for them to do better the things they ought to be doing.

Strictly speaking, if we are considering ineffective rather than just inappropriate treatments, it might be argued that there is no loss of comprehensiveness in eliminating certain treatments from the scope of finance. There is no benefit in the public provision of snake-medicine, and so no loss of comprehensivenss if snake-medicine is not provided. But, as we shall see, things are not quite so simple.

It may prove difficult to identify ineffective treatments or to agree on what is inappropriate.

Let us turn first to the so-called inappropriate treatments. For proponents of the strategy of focused service provision, tattoo removal stands as a paradigm of the sort of thing that publicly assured health care systems ought not to be doing at all; other therapies often mentioned include assisted conception, gender reassignment and breast augmentation.

Perhaps what is intended to bind these rather diverse examples together is that they are all supposed to be cases of desire rather than need. People can live without children or in the gender to which they are born. Of course they may not have as happy a life as if they were able to conceive, or assume a new gender identity, but no one, so the argument continues, has a right to happiness, or at least no one has the right to achieve happiness at the expense of others. Though common, the argument is flawed.

In the first place, it substantially overestimates how much activity in these sorts of categories is currently undertaken by public systems like the NHS. It is very difficult to obtain *in vitro* fertilisation on the NHS, for example, and many of those who receive some health service funding will not receive the full cost of treatment. Of course the procedures crop up frequently in discussion, for the very good reason that they are marginal, and funding allocations are all about what you are to do at the margins. But we are simply fooling ourselves if we think that there are large savings to be made under these headings. Many of the savings are already being made through a process of rationing by denial or delay.

But, even if this were not true, the argument for eliminating the inappropriate therapies rests on too simple a distinction between wants and needs, what it is good for people to have and what it is necessary for them to have. Even in the case of tattoos, for example, you will find cases where tattoo removal is necessary to help prisoners establish themselves in the labour market and reform their lives. And is it really so sensible to be willing to treat the depression brought on by infertility or a sense of embarrassment at some feature of one's appearance but not the underlying condition? Conversely, if we simply say we fund the essentials, what happens to minor quality-of-life interventions, like the removal of ear wax, which no one questions, in the health service?

Moreover, simply to have a blanket ban on certain activities undermines the comprehensiveness principle in another way. If *in vitro* fertilisation or 'cosmetic' surgery is simply eliminated in principle from public systems, it will not mean that such activities are not undertaken; it will simply mean that they will be undertaken privately for those who can afford to pay for them, leaving the rest of the population to their own devices. In this way, treatments that are of marginal cost significance to the system as a whole, but with significant implications for individual patients, will be taken out of the scope of provision.

What about ineffective therapies? Here again, great promise is held out. If only we could get rid of the ineffective therapies, the argument runs, we should be able to release resources for the things that really work. Evidence-based medicine, it is suggested, should replace hunch medicine, and then we shall have enough in the way of resources to do the worthwhile things.

There is no doubt that professionals in all walks of life should strive to make sure that their activities are effective, and I for one welcome the stress in the movement for evidence-based medicine on ensuring that there really is a basis in knowledge of medical alternatives. However, I doubt that it is the panacea to the the problem of resources that its proponents are sometimes wont to suggest, and this for a number of reasons.

In the first place, there may simply not be the evidence available to warrant the denial of certain treatments to individuals. What we are talking about is often professional consensus rather than evidence in any hard sense. Sometimes the professional consensus has sufficient warrant of experience to pass muster as a reasonable basis for treatment and provision. The fact that removal of the appendix in cases of appendicitis has not been warranted by double-blind randomised controlled trial should not put it into the suspect category. Even where this is not so, however, the appeal to evidence may be exaggerated, if it means that health care systems should stop providing certain therapies until evidence of their effectiveness is available. To stop providing something that is thought in good faith to be of benefit, even if no statistical demonstration of the benefit is available, is to pose a very severe test of what may be thought reasonable.

Second, whether something is effective or ineffective is simply not like a light bulb, which is either on or off. Evidence about effectiveness normally comes in a statistical form, showing that a particular treatment or drug regime is effective only in a small proportion of cases. Indeed, this was precisely the sort of issue that was being dealt with in the Jaymee Bowen case, where the question was whether the health authority should finance a second bone marrow transplant in the hope of overcoming her leukaemia. No clinician who was involved in that case thought there was no chance that a second bone-marrow transplant would work: it was rather that the chances were thought to be so low that it was not worth putting the child through the torment of the procedure (Ham and Pickard, 1998, pp. 16–31).

But what is the right figure here? Is a mere 1 in 10 chance sufficient to say that a procedure is ineffective, or does it have to drop to 1 in 100, or 1 in 1,000? It is too simple to say of certain procedures, therefore, that they are simply ineffective, when evidence about their effect takes a statistical form. Moreover, precisely because so much evidence is statistical in character, the problem arises as to how the statistical generalisation is to be applied to the particular. As Marmor and Blustein (1994, p. 96) have pointed out, judging how to proceed in questionable cases is part of what constitutes the art of medicine. But as soon as we concede this degree of discretion we are some distance from the original thought that there could be a blanket identification of certain sorts of therapies that can be excluded from the scope of social insurance cover.

Moreover, as soon as you start to talk about the odds of success you have also to start talking about the cost of even considering the therapy in question. I guess that few of us would have problems with the thought that £10 for a treatment that had a 1 in 10,000 chance of saving a child's life was a good buy. What would we think, however, of £1 million for a 1 in 10,000 chance? In other words, once you start to talk about effectiveness it is difficult not to be talking about cost-effectiveness and we have lost the clear distinction that the original proposal had between those things the NHS should be doing and those things it should not be doing. We can also see how the question passes from a purely technical judgement about effectiveness to an issue of social principle about how much it is worth paying for a certain probability of effectiveness.

If doing nothing is not an option, and identifying a clear class of activities that can be excluded from the scope of public coverage is not an option, then we shall have to think about alternatives. One possible thought to have here is that we should strive to do better with the resources we have at our disposal: the NHS, and similar socialised systems, should become more efficient in the way they use resources. Indeed, so obvious a thought is this that it has even occurred to politicians. We may not be able to get a quart out of a pint pot, but at least we should try to get a pint out of a pint pot, and if we cross our fingers we may even get just a little bit more.

In recent years the search for efficiency savings has been considerable, and has been reflected in higher activity levels within the NHS as well as in schemes like the sale or lease of assets. But how far does it go in solving the problem with which we started?

Just as with the principle of effectiveness, there is always an argument of professional responsibility for seeking to maximise the efficient use of resources. However, the extent to which efficiency gains can solve our initial problem is limited. Higher rates of activity cannot be sustained indefinitely without severe loss of morale and professional esteem. Moreover, the stress upon greater efficiency risks accepting the fallacy of thinking that all members of a group can operate above the average level. To be sure, there are important issues about the balance to be struck between the interests of providers on the one hand and those of patients and taxpayers on the other, but it would be Panglossian to think that all the problems of rationing can be solved merely by introducing suitable incentives for professionals and other providers to become more efficient.

Summarising the discussion so far, then, we can see that modifying the principle of comprehensiveness in such a way as to make it compatible with the requirements of high-quality care available to all without financial barriers is not possible without running into serious problems about the values that would thereby have to be compromised or sacrificed. That being the case, we should now turn to other ways of resolving the conflicts implicit in our original inconsistent triad.

SHOULD PUBLIC SCHEMES DROP THE COMMITMENT TO HIGH-QUALITY CARE?

The notion that comprehensive freely available forms of health care have to sacrifice the quality of care is one that is often found in policy discussions. In accounts of the UK's NHS, it might be called the 'Brookings' critique, after the Washington-based think-tank of that name. In one of its studies (Aaron and Schwartz, 1984) the argument was that the NHS underserves its patients, with too few diagnostic tests, too much waiting, not enough screening and an unwillingness to use expensive therapies.

In a more recent Brookings publication a similar story is told:

> British doctors do not go looking for trouble: if the patient
> does not report symptoms, doctors are unlikely to order

tests on their own. A 1978 study showed that diabetes diagnosis depended more on symptoms, and less on routine testing, in Britain than in India, Poland, France, or East Berlin,
or on an American Indian reservation. British cardiologists
are less likely than Americans to prescribe angiography on
the basis of tests, and more likely to do so in response to
persistence of symptoms after maximum medical therapy.
'You can't be diagnosed as having hypertension if nobody
takes your blood pressure,' Lynn Payer summarizes.
'But,' she adds, 'even when blood pressure is taken, the
British have a higher threshold for disease.'

(White, 1995, p. 123)

Perhaps those war films showing the British as a phlegmatic race
stoically coping with adversity and deprivation were not misleading
after all?

It is of course possible to contest this characterisation in many
ways. In claiming to present instances of a more general characterisation, it conflates high-quality medicine with interventionist
medicine. It does not offer a systematic comparison across a whole
range of medical procedures. And it neglects the strong science bias
of British medicine that leads clinicians to be sceptical of many
fashionable procedures. However, in some ways these objections
are not to the point. The issue is how far there is a sound ethical
basis for the claim that failure to pursue high-quality care is a
fault in a health care system.

In part, the worry about the failure to maintain the quality of care
stems from the same ethical sources as the worries about comprehensiveness and availability. If high quality is not maintained, and
if a private alternative is allowed (as it almost certainly must be),
then a failure of quality in the public system will lead individuals
to exit to the private system, thus reintroducing the inequality of
access that public provision or financing was intended to abolish.
From this point of view there is no distinct moral issue.

However, the matter cannot be laid so quietly to rest. Suppose the
failure of quality is widespread and that it affects not only those who
cannot exit to the private system but also those who can but choose
not to. Suppose, that is to say, that there is a general cultural acceptance of low standards of care. Should this matter?

One reason why it may matter is that it is extremely difficult for
individuals to assess whether the treatment they can expect to receive
within any one system is high-quality or not. This is not a paternal-

istic point which denies that each person is the best judge of his or her own welfare. Rather it is a point about the difficulty of judging the performance of a system in the absence of any comparative experience. Thus I am not saying that if people had experience of both a high-quality system and a low-quality system they would mistake the one for the other. Instead, I am simply noting that the comparison is one that few people are exposed to over a long enough period. Acquiescence in low standards may not mean very much by itself.

However, there is another reason for being concerned about quality. A health care system has responsibilities towards its workers as well as towards it patients. It is inconsistent with those responsibilities to ask professionals to work in a system in which they cannot practise to a high standard. It is asking them to suppress what should be a central element of the motivation that their training has instilled within them. We do not have to be unduly Aristotelean to think that the practitioners of an art need to be able to aim towards excellence. In other words, the sacrifice of quality is not an easy option.

CONCLUSION

Our inconsistent triad remains, therefore. There is a tension among the three elements of the basic principle of modern health care, but it is not possible to resolve it by simply dropping one of the elements. We seem to have a built-in contradiction. But conflicts of value are not like conflicts of belief (cf. Williams, 1973, pp. 166–86). In the first place, when two beliefs conflict, coming to see the truth of one normally entails seeing the falsity of the other. Conflicts of value are not like that: in discovering that comprehensiveness is important in a health care system, we do not thereby see that high-quality care is less important. Second, choosing to hold to a belief typically tends to weaken the grip of the contradictory belief. Not so with values, where choosing a policy in line with one value leaves one with a sense of regret for values not pursued.

Indeed, conflicts of value are typical in all fields of public policy: between economic growth and environmental protection; between individual freedom and social stability; between humanitarian intervention and recognising the right of national self-determination; between comprehensiveness, quality and availability in health care. As Sir Isaiah Berlin (1969, p. 171) argued many years ago, human goals are many, and in perpetual rivalry with one another. To suppose otherwise is to cast a metaphysical blanket over self-deceit or hypocrisy. To suppose otherwise in the field of health care is to do less than justice to the achievements that the socialisation of health care represents.

REFERENCES

Aaron, H. and Schwartz, W. B. (1984) *The Painful Prescription: Rationing Hospital Care* (Washington, D.C.: Brookings Institution).

Berlin, I. (1969) *Four Essays on Liberty* (Oxford: Oxford University Press).

Ham, C. and Pickard, S. (1998) *Tragic Choices in Health Care: The Case of Child B* (London: King's Fund).

Heidenheimer, A. J., Heclo, H. and Adams, C. T. (1990) *Comparative Public Policy* (New York: St Martin's Press).

Klein, R., Day, P. and Redmayne, S. (1996) *Managing Scarcity* (Buckingham: Philadelphia).

Marmor, T. and Blustein, J. (1994) 'Cutting waste by making rules: promises, pitfalls, and realistic prospects' in T. R. Marmor, *Understanding Health Care Reform* (New Haven and London: Yale University Press), pp. 86–106.

Reinhardt, U. E. (1987) 'Resource allocation in health care: the allocation of lifestyles to providers', *Milbank Quarterly* 65: 2, pp. 153–76.

Schumpeter, J. (1942) *Capitalism, Socialism and Democracy* (London: Allen & Unwin).

Weale, A. (1995) 'The Ethics of Rationing', *British Medical Bulletin* 51: 4, pp. 831–41.

White, J. (1995) *Competing Solutions* (Washington, D.C.: Brookings Institution).

Williams, B. (1973) *Problems of the Self* (Cambridge: Cambridge University Press).

Williamson, O. E. (1986) *Economic Organisation* (Brighton: Harvester-Wheatsheaf).

8

MORE PRIVATE HEALTH INSURANCE IS DESIRABLE AND INEVITABLE

David Cavers

Ask people in the UK about the NHS in the abstract, and many will tell you that it is a wonderful institution, the envy of the world. Ask them about their own real life experiences, or those of their family and friends, and their enthusiasm becomes more measured. Ask those people who have experience of both the NHS and various overseas systems of health care delivery (including foreigners' views) and the envy is simply not in evidence. People in certain other countries believe they now manage these things decidedly better than we do.

When it comes to *private* health care, appalling stories of failings in the US system usually emerge as dire portents of how things would develop in the UK if the private sector were to take hold here. Such stories may sometimes indeed be true, but they are usually retold by those seeking to make a political point and are rarely accompanied by any balanced reporting of the successes of American health care. In any event, for most people who work in the UK private sector, the American system is as remote from their ambition as it could be. Much more desirable are the mixed economies found elsewhere around the developed world, where high-quality health care is routinely delivered without the political and commercial criticisms so often applied to health care in the UK and the US. Our national system and the American national system are at opposite ends of a spectrum, and both fail many of their citizens.

In this chapter I argue that we need to adapt health care delivery in Britain in order to achieve higher levels of health gain, as well as greater economic efficiency of process. Such outcomes will not be achievable without the commitment of much greater amounts of money than are now being spent. It is unlikely that they will come from government, and, in my view, it is much better if they come from private purses. The existing private sector in the UK (still less that of the US) is not a model for the future, but a genuine mixed economy of the kind found elsewhere in the world most certainly is. Why, and how, this should be raises a variety of ethical issues which are flagged and offered for debate.

It will come as no surprise that someone who works in the independent sector should champion a market approach. There are market disciplines which have been tested and developed across the range of human endeavour and there is no earthly reason to suppose that health care is so unique as to be kept immune from them. What is more, the market approach is compatible with a social duty to ensure that treatment not be withheld simply because of inability to pay. Indeed, around the developed world all governments (including those in North America) spend around 5 per cent of their national income on state-funded health care, and this money provides varying degrees of 'safety-net' provision. The difference between the UK and almost everywhere else in the world is that, whilst we limit ourselves to what is seemingly a universal, government-paid and organised safety net only, other countries also have a significant private contribution of monies (another 3 per cent or so of GDP) to add to their government's expenditure. It is this which marks their higher public satisfaction levels – and arguably better health outcomes than our own (see below).

In the UK system, people seem almost to pride themselves on working to a lowest common denominator in health care provision (inevitable where everyone has equal access to care but overall funds are tightly limited), rather than seeking higher standards driven upwards by a greater degree of selectivity. However, such 'market mechanisms' as now exist in the UK are restricted to a somewhat economically inefficient private sector, and to an internal market, introduced in the 1990s into the NHS, but which is still solidly driven by supply-side rather than demand considerations. One good question about such a form of delivery is this. How can the customer's voice truly be heard when the person who decides how much health care the NHS will give you, or me, or anybody else, is the Chancellor of the Exchequer? For it is the Chancellor who sets the NHS's annual budget each year on the basis of successful bidding or otherwise from the various competing Secretaries of

State of the day. And it is that total NHS budget which produces the rationing of care which runs down the bureaucratic line to individual clinicians having to make competing judgements about individual patients' needs. For we do, indeed, require our doctors to be expert in rationing. Patients do not make their job any easier. Not only is health care provided to them free at the point of use but they are encouraged in the belief that they have an inalienable right to use it. In such a climate patients cannot be expected to make the sort of efficient use of that service that is commonplace when payments pass from one hand to another. On the contrary, the 'normal' basis of judgement – price – is completely absent from most health care decisions. Our NHS system therefore requires doctors to manage primarily from a supply-side consideration, and 'demand' is, to all intents and purposes, managed by restricting availability either in time (to produce, for example, waiting lists) or in space (to restrict, for example, the number of available beds and, increasingly, the kinds of treatment which the public sector is prepared to offer).

What one finds in the NHS, then, is something less than adherence to a market approach; and the existing private sector in the UK is not an altogether effective market model either. It, too, has various economic inefficiencies within it as a result of monopolistic practices by its providers (of which more anon) which keep prices high. If the independent sector is to make progress, if a mixed economy is to become a much more real possibility, such monopolies will have to be broken.

So this chapter speculates on growing the private element of medicine, and yet also on controlling its cost, with the aim of producing better health care for all.

THE NHS BACKGROUND

A short historical digression will help to set the stage. Since its foundation in 1948, in the space of less than a generation, most of the citizens of the UK have become enthusiastic users and supporters of the NHS. Through the NHS they have come to enjoy comprehensive health care free at the point of use.

The NHS took the place of a mixed economy of voluntary, public and private arrangements where those who could afford to do so had been expected to contribute financially to their care. Care was not exactly denied if a patient could not afford to pay, but the extent of that care was usually related to the payment that was made.

General practitioners charged for their services and were remunerated from 'panel' membership or by out-of-pocket payment. In hospitals, almoners assessed patients' ability to pay. Working people, urged on by their trade unions, joined friendly societies or Saturday funds which effectively gave insurance cover against such costs. The middle classes, left to their own devices, joined local provident associations to the same end. Health care thus operated in a commercial market place much like any other. If you were insured, or could afford to pay, you were treated; if not, too bad.

As a system, it was criticised for its part in contributing to the five giant evils identified by Beveridge as afflicting the core of the nation and standing in need of major reform (Disease, Squalor, Want, Ignorance and Idleness) – which led to the creation of the modern welfare state. If only, it was argued, the supposed chronic pool of disease perpetuated by the old system could be eradicated by a new comprehensive and free service, health care would play its part in effecting a giant social leap forward.

And so the NHS came into being. In theory, the insurance mechanisms which had supported the earlier system should have become redundant, since care was no longer a matter of affordability. But public trust in new approaches is rarely universal, and survive such mechanisms did, with the provident insurers in particular adapting their place in the system to a new and revised rationale.

WHY GO PRIVATE?

For many, the ability to choose where and when, and by whom, to be treated counted for a great deal. To have the relative peace and comfort of a pay-bed, or a single room in one of the remaining charitable hospitals, was important. And, most significantly, the emerging waiting lists within NHS hospital services as the system failed to realise the (in retrospect incredibly naive) expectation of eradicating disease became a strong motivator to acquiring private medical insurance as a means of affording quicker care.

So whereas, prior to 1948, everyone was required to pay and the care they received was largely undifferentiated, after 1948 payment came to be associated with a means of avoiding the drawbacks of the universal health care delivery service. Private health care runs along similar lines still. People in the UK buy private medical insurance (or pay for *ad hoc* treatment from their own pockets) in order to have speedier access to secondary (hospital) care which would otherwise be essentially 'free' altogether from the NHS.

Most customers of private medical insurance have no similar motivation at primary care (GP) level. They have been perfectly prepared to utilise the universal NHS GP service, which they have perceived as working satisfactorily to their own advantage, but not the NHS hospital service, which they sometimes regard as poor.

In this they are aided and abetted by the structures within which the medical profession works. Access by the public to GPs is relatively easy; access to consultants is closely controlled, and visits are rare; consultants' time is provided only at a premium (which in particular has spawned the secretive NHS merit awards system as well as an inflated private fee structure).

Private medicine today is not cheap. Much of the existing market rests on employers providing various of their employees with private medical insurance as a fringe benefit. And it is readily apparent that purchasing by individuals (as opposed to employers) is closely correlated to trends in real disposable incomes and consumer spending at large. As a voluntary purchase item – and an aspirational one at that – private medical insurance competes with other goods and services for its share of family expenditure. As disposable incomes rise, so does the extent of coverage of private medical insurance. But when times are tough – and 'feel good' is widely lacking – the market remains flat.

Today's private health sector, then, is the result of two major factors – disenchantment with one part (a very large and critical part) of the NHS; and a desire to use rising levels of affluence to improve health care quality at the margin for oneself and one's family. It has not been driven principally by ideology (although there is a close relationship between buying private medical insurance and broader lifestyle choices that have right-of-centre political associations), nor have people opted for private medical insurance expecting significantly better care. There is widespread confidence in the ability of doctors and nurses, whether they are working in the public or in the private sector, and few people would expect the care itself somehow to be 'worse' in the public sphere.

At a time when self-provision is increasingly expected as a major means of funding many welfare benefits, what, if anything, is ethically wrong with self-funded medical care? Isn't the trend already established in optical services, for example? Not without regular and on-going criticism, admittedly, these services, which now need to be purchased privately, are widely if grudgingly accepted. Or take dentistry. People pay for private dentists principally because they cannot find a dentist prepared to put them on his/her NHS list – not because private treatment is supposed to be more skilful. (As a *post hoc* rationalisation this may well emerge, of course – payment tends to equate with an expectation of value – but it is not a critical aspect to the initial decision to 'go private'). In any event, NHS dentistry is far from free, other than for children and specified groups of adults. The rest of us already pay significantly towards the total cost of treatment.

HOW TO FUND THE HEALTH CARE WE NEED

To shift the argument from the individual to the macro level, we need to examine our health care system within the context of total demand and the state's ability to fund it. Such issues really are vital to the future nature of health care in Britain.

The NHS represents a major component of the welfare state. It consumed £39 billion in 1995 – £700 for each man, woman and child in the country. It is hardly 'free'. But the NHS budget is, of course, only one element of government spending and it competes for monies with every other sector. The three big welfare departments of state – Health, Social Services and Education – together consume over 60 per cent of public sector expenditure. Each has heavyweight proponents arguing for higher levels of expenditure, which in many instances (much of social services, for example) represent mandatory payments rather than discretionary ones.

Spending on the NHS has recently been increasing in real terms, but as a proportion of national income there has been little movement in the 1990s. It is difficult to see how this might change in future. Governments in the developed world appear to be committed to a maximum tax take not exceeding 40 per cent of their country's GDP (the UK is currently at 42 per cent), and indeed John Major as Prime Minister aimed over the long term at a rate of 35 per cent.

Where, then, is additional funding to come from for the Welfare State and for the NHS within it – always assuming that greater spending on such services is a good thing (of which more later)? Clearly the latest NHS reforms have represented a serious attempt to remedy supply-side inefficiencies. 'More' money can come from obtaining better value from what is spent, from greater productivity, from limiting the service to what is necessary rather than perhaps merely desired. (I distinguish between what an individual may 'desire' and what a medical professional may believe to be 'desirable'. The public, for example, may expect a prescription for an antibiotic for every respiratory illness, which a doctor most certainly will not prescribe.)

MORE PRIVATE SPENDING

If people 'bought' health care as they do any other goods or services, what shape would 'demand' take, and what would the resulting health gain look like? Certainly, people's expectations of their health care system, ill informed though many of them are, are for ever rising. The rise is based upon a combination of medical advances enabling more to be done and people's wish to benefit accordingly – from dramatic things like transplant surgery to the routine. An enormous number of hip replacements are now done, which twenty years ago were still largely experimental. Then there is the health gain – measurable in quality as well as quantity of years – due to drug treatment for such things as hypertension, chronic chest diseases and childhood illnesses. When such treatments become available, should not all our citizens have access to the cure or the relief of symptoms which is promised?

As medicine can do more, people will want more. And in so far as their quality of life is improving in other directions as living standards rise, why should they not want greater attention to all their health care needs? Paying for these demands will involve going well beyond the expenditure which is determined for them by their professional medical attendants acting under budgetary orders from the Chancellor of the Exchequer. Almost inevitably, the answer has to lie in greater private provision, but not necessarily private provision as we currently understand it. It can be expected to have a public element as well, and so to belong to a more mixed economy than we have at present.

Such a conclusion is not limited, of course, to the needs of the country's health services. It applies to the whole of the welfare state. Indeed, in other areas the government has already taken action to encourage private provision – such as in occupational and personal pensions as an alternative to the State Earnings Related Pensions Scheme. Tax relief on contributions to personally and privately funded pensions is a major motivator. We have seen state incapacity benefits limited to below subsistence level, whilst at the same time payments under income protection insurance policies have been made available tax-free as an incentive to take out the alternative of private cover. And the country is engaged in a broad debate about how to pay for residential and nursing care in old age – not a burden which the state wishes to shoulder, since the projected costs are staggering.

The economic arguments look compelling. If government is unwilling to tax beyond a given limit (if it does it probably will not be re-elected) but the population wants a whole range of yet more extensive and expensive welfare benefits, the only alternative source of payment (in whole or in part) is private pockets. Many forms of private provision are possible. But what seems most equitable is an arrangement which encourages a mixed economy of public and private contributions, rather than a complete break between the two that might have serious overtones of social division. Examples of such approaches from elsewhere in the world appear to deliver greater benefit, and it is worth taking a moment or two to consider them.

THE INTERNATIONAL SCENE

On any international comparison, at least with the rest of the developed world, the UK devotes amongst the lowest of all percentages of its national income to health care. The advocates of the present system argue that this reflects administrative efficiency; its detractors say that it indicates a level of unmet demand which is, in its own way, inimical to higher levels of macro-economic performance. Interestingly, most countries spend 6–7 per cent of their national income on health care from public resources. The wide variations in total spending come about from the significantly greater private contributions found elsewhere in the world (see Table 8.1).

Table 8.1 Health expenditure as a percentage of GDP

Country	Public	Private	Total
US	7.6	8.1	15.7
Canada	7.2	2.7	9.9
France	6.8	2.4	9.2
Germany	6.0	2.5	8.5

Source: OECD, 1994.

The value achieved by these differential levels of spending is not easy to determine, because it is difficult to produce any simplified index of benefit from health spending. The public would like to believe that there are readily quantifiable states of 'being well' or 'being ill', the latter leading to explicit requirements for the use of medical services. But health is not at all like that. There are, of course, various conditions which we can all agree constitute 'illness' and which call for medical intervention. They range from the life-threatening to the relatively straightforward, in clinical terms at least (such as meningitis and malignant cancers on the one hand and bronchitis and cysts on the other), but what of that vast army of other calls on health services that result in significant costs but seemingly no tangible gain? What of all those hysterectomies, D-and-Cs and tonsillectomies which used to be carried out wholesale not so very long ago but which are now regarded – at least in statistical, whole population, terms – as being of questionable value as surgical fashion changes? And what of hip operations, which used to require patients to be seriously immobilised by pain before treatment took place, as against the tendency nowadays for much earlier intervention? How do we summarise all this into some more readily and comprehensively understood criteria of health gain?

Different answers to this question are given in different parts of the world. One study examined a series of health indices and presented answers on each public's satisfaction with its health care system as a means of making such a comparison (see Table 8.2). An absolute conclusion on what is right and what is wrong with each country's approach is hard to define from the results, except that (the US apart) there is a positive correlation between higher levels of spending and higher levels of public satisfaction. Such a conclusion should not in general be a matter of surprise, but to the British public, accustomed to believe that its national health service is the envy of the world, it comes as something of a shock to discover that other countries may actually be doing it better. If, as I have been arguing, UK spending on health provision must also come to a greater extent from private rather than public sources, what issues arise for ethical debate? Is an individual's (privately paid for) health gain to be deprecated because a fellow citizen fails to achieve a similar advantage from a publicly funded system? And what are the responsibilities of the professionals in the system, accustomed to managing principally from supply-side considerations (i.e. their own), rather than from those of their patients? These are questions I raise rather than answer.

Table 8.2 Public satisfaction and expenditure levels

	Public satisfaction (%)	Health care expenditure per capita ($)
Canada	56	1,795
Netherlands	47	1,182
France	41	1,379
Germany	41	1,287
Sweden	32	1,421
Japan	29	1,113
UK	27	909
Spain	21	730
Italy	12	1,113
US	10	2,566

Source: National Economic Research Associates, May 1993.
Note: Health care expenditures are based on purchasing power parities, using notional exchange rates derived from the prices of a representative bundle of goods and services in each country.

MANAGED CARE

Now for some concrete examples of developments in the mixed economy of health care. To begin with, considerable resources are being devoted by private medical insurers and others to evaluating 'managed care'. Managed care is a matter of the insurer (or whoever is responsible for purchasing, as opposed to receiving, the care) insisting on introducing an efficiency dimension into the clinical decisions reached by doctor and patient.

That such a move could come from the private sector of medicine, where freedom of choice for the patient has long been the battle cry, may seem odd. It is the NHS which shackles doctors' good intentions by persistent reminders of budgetary constraints, requiring the use of cheaper drug equivalents and early discharge so as to free beds for the next round of patients, not the private sector. In a market-driven system where the customer is paramount, should not the customer and his/her representative (the doctor) decide what is required rather than some third party seeking to interfere in that process?

What we have at the moment, even in the private sector, is a system largely unfettered by commercial considerations of real economic value. Suppliers – doctors and hospitals – have both been characterised in official reports as acting in highly monopolistic ways. The very structure of UK private medicine has resulted in high costs for private care, and high premiums for private medical insurance schemes. The question of how to limit these costs, reduce premiums and attract significantly larger numbers of customers is the crucial one for all private medical insurers. Everyone wants the same volumes of care for less money, or more care for the same money: managed care offers the prospect of a significant way forward.

So what is managed care? It comes in many forms in those parts of the world where it is already practised (principally so far in North America), but in essence it allows the insurer a say in what, where and how treatment takes place in an effort to reduce costs. It emphatically does not put the insurer into a clinical decision-making role, but it does give him a much bigger voice in the treatment plan. Take a typical referral as it happens at present. A GP tells his patient a hip replacement may be needed and refers him to an orthopaedic surgeon. Currently, the surgeon sees the patient, agrees the operation, carries it out and sends the patient home before anyone has enquired about the costs. In future, the insurer will have agreed with the self-same orthopaedic surgeon in advance a best practice protocol which determines the criteria for admission, the treatment plan and the discharge arrangements, as well as all medical and hospital charges. There are two emphases in the plan – higher-quality care, but at lower overall cost. A further step might be to limit the number of orthopaedic surgeons whom the insurer is prepared to 'recognise', and the hospitals at which such treatment can take place – again in exchange for sizeable price reductions as a result of such 'preferred provider' volume-based deals.

This time, our patient (or his GP) telephones the insurer before any referral takes place. The insurer agrees the choice of specialist and hospital, and talks to both about the implementation of the protocol for the patient. All the details are agreed in advance, including an appreciably lower bill than would otherwise have been the case.

Is everyone happy? The patient gets treated in accordance with best-practice protocols; the surgeon and the hospital get larger volumes of patients by way of preferred provider arrangements; the insurer gets lower prices (and much less administrative hassle in settling bills after the event, because they have all been prior agreed). Most important, costs are reduced and premiums for medical insurance can therefore be lower, so the market may be stimulated to expand.

If this all sounds too pat, consider what managed care activities in the US have achieved. Numbers of bed-days per 1,000 patients have been more than halved in comparison with traditional arrangements, with no discernible reduction in the quality of outcomes. Indeed, the concentration on what currently constitutes 'best practice', and its dissemination around the country, help to ensure that every specialised unit comes closer to being a centre of excellence. In the meantime, the cost reductions are passed on to customers by way of premium rate adjustments.

THE PAY-BED REVOLUTION

Getting doctors to compete with each other via preferred-provider dealing is one means of improving efficiency in the existing private sector. Another is to encourage competition amongst hospitals. This is less easy than it seems. Most patients prefer to be treated locally – the country simply does not travel to Harley Street for its care, even if people like to think of the private sector in such a way – and, outside London, most private hospitals face little by way of local competition. One answer lies in encouraging local pay-bed units to compete with them. There have always been private patients in NHS hospitals. When hospitals were nationalised after 1948, the co-operation of the consultant body was ensured by allowing consultants to continue to treat private patients in pay-beds specifically authorised for the purpose in NHS hospitals. For twenty years, pay-beds provided the principal means of private treatment.

The Labour government in the late 1970s tried to abolish pay-beds. It failed, but its efforts so frightened the provident associations that they set about encouraging independent hospital building. As a result, pay-beds' share of the market dropped like a stone to not much more than 10 per cent in the late 1980s.

The NHS reforms of the early 1990s allowed hospital trusts to begin to generate income by competing vigorously again for private patients. By 1995 their share of such patients had improved to 16 per cent, and at least one commentator has speculated that, taken together, they could within a year or two again become the largest single provider of private patient activity. A real renaissance for pay-beds.

Is this ethical behaviour? The question is valid from two perspectives in particular – first, should the NHS be treating private patients at all; and second, is it offering fair competition to the independent hospitals?

In answering the first point, we need to bear in mind that no one, by opting to pay, is deprived of the right to the same free NHS treatment as any other citizen; by choosing private care, that patient leaves more money in the system for treating others who remain within an NHS ambit. It is quite clear nowadays that this is the major limiting factor on NHS care. It is not the physical availability of individual doctors, nurses and equipment, but simply whether or not the funds are available to pay for their services, which determines the volume of treatment activity which takes place.

Is it then ethical for such private treatment to take place in an NHS, rather than an independent, hospital? There seems to me to be no logical reason why not. No NHS patient is disadvantaged – as we have seen, waiting lists exist because of budgetary constraints, not because a surgeon or nurse is away dealing with private patients. In any event, if the NHS makes a profit from private patient work, such funds are available to add to the NHS pot. One might indeed argue that, since there is an absolute requirement on the NHS to provide care for everyone free at the point of use, any charges which it does make to some patients at the margin actually represent a desirable improvement in its financial position and should be welcomed accordingly.

The second question – is such competition fair, or is the NHS abusing its ability to offer lower-priced care than the independent hospital down the road – has been comprehensively answered in Davies et al. (1995). Not only is the competition honourable, it also produces worthwhile profits for the NHS to put into public care needs.

Competition is a nice kind of answer to a number of ethical issues. It ensures that the NHS does what it is required to do, and is good at doing, given the appropriate funding – i.e. delivering quality clinical care. It enables patients, who by and large feel an affinity for, and a desire to support, their local NHS hospital, to be treated at that hospital but to standards and times more of their choosing than the Treasury's. It enables doctors to work with private as well as public patients on the same campus without the one detracting from the other in terms of the consultant's ready availability should an acute need arise. It gives medical insurers (and hence their customers) more competitive rates than would otherwise be on offer. And it demonstrates that a mixed economy in health care – public and private provision side by side – can work sensibly, enhancing the total amount of health care available to the community as a whole.

CONCLUSION

These, then, are some of the issues for the private sector today:

- Should people have to pay more themselves for higher standards of care, or should the tax bill rise in order to provide the necessary funds?
- Should market mechanisms be more strongly developed in health care delivery?
- Should medical insurers act on patients' behalf in introducing managed care techniques to raise efficiency amongst providers?
- And should pay-bed units be expanded on NHS campuses, with an aim of producing profit to be ploughed back into public health care?

My answer is yes to each of these. As a result the UK will enjoy a much stronger health care system, to the undoubted benefit of all its citizens.

REFERENCE

Davies, K., Booer, T. and Lewis, D. (1995) *Are Pay-beds Profitable?* London: National Economic Research Associates.

9

EQUAL ACCESS TO HEALTH CARE

A problematic ideal

Will Cartwright

The notion that there should be equal access to health care seems to command very wide support in the UK and may be thought to be the animating principle of the NHS. Indeed, in Chapter 7 of this volume Albert Weale argues that, despite the heterogeneity of the institutional structures for delivering health care in the Western democracies, those structures are all broadly consistent with the requirement of equal access, except in the United States. He calls this requirement 'the basic principle of modern health care organisation'.[1] However, the fact that a principle is basic is no guarantee that its form is perspicuous, as philosophers know discouragingly well. In this case there are both contentious issues about how to formulate the principle and conceptual obscurities about some of its constituent notions. The need to come to grips with these problems assumes a particular urgency at present in the light of the shortage of resources for health care[2] and of proposals to overcome it by greater use of private funds,[3] both of which may be thought to constitute threats to the principle of equal access. I propose to review some of these problems and to relate the results to the suggestions of Weale and of David Cavers, another contributor to this volume.[4]

ACCESS AND EQUALITY

The two key notions in the principle, access and equality, are both problematic. While in some cases a judgement about equal access

165

can be made readily enough, in others it is less clear whether access is equal or indeed what counts as an issue of access.

Equality

We can agree, presumably, that the denial of medical care on the grounds of religion, race, political belief or social position constitutes a lack of equal access. But in the Western democracies it is money rather than these factors that is more usually the topic of concern in discussions of access. Once again it is widely supposed that access is not equal if some people are denied care because they cannot afford it. By contrast the bearing of age on the distribution of health care engenders more controversy. In so far as the elderly are denied a treatment because their prospects of benefiting from it are very slim, this should not be regarded as a denial of equal access if younger patients similarly unlikely to benefit are also denied the treatment. For in that case it is not age, but likelihood of benefit, that is the ground of the decision. If, however, the treatment is withheld from the elderly on what one might call efficiency grounds, because, though it might be successful, it would yield fewer life years than if applied to younger patients who may be expected to live longer, then that should be deemed a denial of equal access to the elderly. For here it is the age of the elderly and their necessarily foreshortened future that steers the decision rather than their clinical prospects. Though it is plain that denying medical care on the basis of age constitutes a case of unequal access, it may be and has been argued that it is nevertheless not unjust, that the access arrangement, though unequal, is not inequitable. Thus it is sometimes said that in the distribution of scarce life-saving therapy those who have already enjoyed the normal span of life, however that is to be construed, should take second place to those who have not yet completed such a span.

Other cases raise difficulties of a different kind. Suppose that there is differential medical provision between town and country, such that physician–patient ratios are more favourable in the cities than in the countryside. Here access seems clearly unequal and, presumably, inequitable. But now suppose that the ratios are equal, but that those in the country have to travel on average further than their urban counterparts in order to reach medical facilities. Is that a case of unequal access? The answer is, I think, far less clear here than in the earlier cases. Or is access unequal if some have on average to wait much longer before they get to see their GP than others?

Or again, to take an example from David Cavers, is access unequal if London commuters have in effect to take half a day off work to see their GP because surgery hours are not accommodated to their patterns of work, whereas the unemployed experience no such inconvenience?[5] These cases differ from the earlier ones to do with race, money, age, and so forth, because in those cases we are standardly talking about the denial of treatment altogether on these grounds, whereas in the present cases the medical service is just more difficult to access, rather than denied outright. In judging whether or not there is equality of access in these cases our intuition fails us, I think. What we can perhaps say more confidently is that the more serious the discrepancy the more likely we are to construe access as unequal, particularly if, as may not be the case, the take-up or use of medical facilities is thereby affected.

Access

The cases that we have just been considering indicate an indefiniteness in the notion of equality as applied in this context. In other cases it is the notion of access that comes under pressure. If a cultural group within a society has a more austere and stoical attitude towards illness than other citizens, such that its members are less inclined to consult doctors, is access here unequal? Is it unequal if some people just dislike doctors and therefore are loath to consult them? Some, I think, are inclined to regard access as here unequal if the cultural and individual attitudes involved are thought of as inhibiting factors that prevent the group or individuals in question from seeking medical help when it is in their supposed interests to do so. This seems to me to be a mistake. The factors involved in these cases are internal psychological ones, having to do with the attitudes of groups or individuals, as distinct from external factors like money or distance that were involved in the earlier cases. There is good reason to regard such internal psychological factors as not bearing upon the notion of access at all.

In order to see this we have to excavate the moral and metaphysical foundations of the concern for equal access. Underlying that concern may be thought to be a conception of human beings as creatures capable of reflecting upon and forming their goals and of choosing and acting accordingly, a conception of them in short as autonomous choosers. Naturally allied with this metaphysical conception of ourselves is a moral concern to respect, and to facilitate the implementation of, these autonomous choices.

External factors that frustrate these choices will then naturally be an object of moral concern. With respect to choices that seem peculiarly vital, such as a decision to seek health care, it will then be morally important to secure access to the objects of such choices, and to do so equally, given that as autonomous choosers human beings may be thought to be equal.

These foundations supply an intelligible rationale for excluding internal psychological factors from the scope of access. A concern for access does not so much encompass such factors as presuppose them. Given certain desires and choices, securing access is about removing external obstacles to their satisfaction and implementation. In the absence of such obstacles variations in the strength of the desire do not affect the equality of access. Those who have the desire only weakly or not at all may be said to have as much access to its object as those who have a strong desire for it. Thus the fact that groups and individuals may vary significantly in their disposition to consult doctors has no bearing upon whether or not they have equal access to medical care.

What will perhaps make such dispositions relevant to access is if they can be represented as psychological blocks making it either impossible or very difficult for the person to satisfy a genuine desire for health. For in this situation the disabling psychological factors begin to assume a status external to the person's self and so, in terms of the above account, can at a pinch be thought to bear upon access. But we cannot just assume that the psychological factors in question are disabling; that needs to be shown. To suppose, in the absence of showing this, that such groups or individuals lack equal access to health care, and to think that their attitudes must then be altered in order to secure it, will constitute both a misunderstanding of access and a moral impertinence.

Access *v.* use

What may tempt some to regard this last class of cases, as well as the previous one, as examples of lack of equal access is the fact, if it is one, that the various factors involved in them lead to differential use of medical care. If differing cultural and individual attitudes, or differing distances from medical facilities and varying times to access them, lead to differing rates of use of them, that will strike many as a matter of concern calling for intervention. This concern with use as distinct from access invites reflection upon the relationship between the two and upon the independent significance of use in assessing the distribution of health care.

If our concern is with access to health care, then use of it is relevant as evidence of access. Discrimination in the distribution of health care may be enshrined in law, in which case its existence is obvious. But there can, of course, be discrimination of an informal kind that is not legally validated and its existence may be harder to establish. One way to do so is to collect evidence about levels of use of health care in different groups. Thus if it is suggested that there is racial discrimination in the distribution of health care, one could test this by comparing the levels of use of health care in the two racial groups, given that the levels of health need in the two groups are similar. But use, it needs to be remembered, is no more than evidence of access, and it is not decisive evidence at that. If use is found to be unequal, that may indicate unequal access, but it need not. For the culture of one of the racial groups may embody different attitudes to health care which cause it to seek it less, and that as we have seen does not make access unequal. Equally, if the use is found to be equal, that may indicate equal access, but arguably it need not. If, despite equal utilisation rates between the two groups, one group has nevertheless to travel further or wait longer to obtain medical attention, then there is at least an argument, as we have seen, for saying that access is not equal.

But sometimes a concern with levels of use seems to reveal an interest in it in its own right, and not just as evidence of access. This is the best way to interpret some responses to those cases where differences of cultural and individual attitude towards medicine lead to differential use of it. As we have seen, such differences cannot be plausibly thought of as indicating unequal access. If moral anxiety about these cases nevertheless survives this conclusion, we may infer that what animates it is an aspiration different from, and more robust than, equal access, to the effect that society should endeavour to engineer equal use of a resource so vital as medical care. Hard on the heels of this aspiration is likely to follow a yet more robust one. Why stop at equal use of medical care? Why not demand equal health outcomes from it? Much depends here upon how we understand the constituent ideas in these aspirations, but notionally one could have equal use that did not lead to equal health outcomes and unequal use that did. In both cases, many will think that it is the outcomes rather than the use that matter. And, finally, most ambitious of all, why limit our concern to equal outcomes from medical treatment when we could aspire to equal health generally? This ideal encompasses, as the others have not, not merely equality in health care roughly speaking, but also equality in the conditions of health, such as diet, housing, even genetic endowment in so far as we are capable of interfering with it. Thus when people complain that there is more ill health among the working class than among others, they are not normally making a point about access to health care. Such discrepancies in health may indicate unequal access, but even if access turned out to be equal, the complaint would still survive because it springs from an aspiration to secure equal health between the classes as an outcome.

As we have seen, the ideal of equal access plausibly presupposes a view of human beings as autonomous choosers and an allied morality of respect for choice. The alternative ideals for medical care and health described in the last paragraph seem to rest upon a different conception of human beings, as social products whose characteristics may therefore be brought within the scope of social control. Those who think that what is important is equal access to health care will be content as long as access is equal, even if people choose to use health care to different degrees. That, it will be said, is their choice, and their choice is to be respected, even if others have doubts about its wisdom. Those, by contrast, who are not content with such different use, and who wish to ensure equal use of medical care, thereby reveal that they view people's choices and behaviour as socially created phenomena that can be engineered for the common good. And the aspirations to secure equal health outcomes from health care use, and more generally to secure equal health, seem to reflect the same conception of human beings.

As we have seen, the ideal of equal health ranges beyond an attempt to equalise the outcome of health care to encompass a concern to equalise the conditions of health, such as housing, diet and even genetics. A similar contrast between access and outcome ideals can be drawn with respect to the conditions of health as was drawn above with respect to health care. The ideal of equal health is committed to equalising as far as possible the conditions of health, whereas an access ideal here would be satisfied by securing to people equal access to these conditions. Contemporary debates about diet and health both illuminate, and are illuminated by, this contrast. For those who adhere to an access ideal it will be important that people are informed as to what is a healthy diet and have the means to secure it. If despite such access they choose like many in Britain to continue to eat an unhealthy diet, that is their affair and their choice is to be respected. Others, including some of the more enthusiastic members of the medical profession, do not share this approach. Perhaps some of these people manage piously to persuade themselves that the widespread persistence of poor diet is due to continuing ignorance and expense. While this is perhaps part of the explanation, it seems extraordinarily hard to believe that it is the whole of it. But what ultimately underlies the determination to press on beyond mere access to a good diet to ensure that, if possible, everyone has a good diet is the vision of human beings as socially created entities, whose features, choices and behaviour can be engineered in their own interest.

The contrast between the access and outcome ideals of health care is thus grounded in a fundamental philosophical debate about the credentials of rival conceptions of human beings, a debate that I cannot explore here.[6]

EQUAL ACCESS TO WHAT?

Beyond the problems posed by the notions of equality and access, there is the fundamental issue of formulating what there is to be equal access to. Simply saying that there must be equal access to health care just serves to conceal the problems. Beginning at the more ambitious end of the possibilities, it might be suggested that there should be equal access to the best possible medical care. If we construe this as something more than the best *available* medical care, it soon becomes apparent how demanding the proposal is, once we remind ourselves that, by spending vastly more on medical research and treatment than we do, we could probably develop and provide treatments way beyond our present capacities. At the limit, of course, this version of the equal access principle, as baldly stated, will be economically unsustainable, but even if we bolt on a qualification of the principle to exclude this danger, the principle in this form is still going to be unacceptable, because it will require a massive diversion of resources from other areas of human activity that we value, starving them unacceptably. Let us then revert to the suggestion briefly alluded to above, to the effect that access should be to the best *available* medical care. Though less demanding than the first proposal, it remains vulnerable to the same two objections and another one.

Imagine that in due course the artificial heart is developed to the point of clinical viability, but that it is immensely expensive to install. To insist upon equal access to this treatment for the vast number who may be thought to need it would once more either be economically unsustainable or at least drain unacceptably large funds from other areas of human activity. Moreover this version of the principle, with its emphasis upon available treatment, omits an issue that the first version at least had the merit of raising, namely whether sufficient funds are being spent, and spent equitably, on the search for new treatments. If we pass now from this demanding end of the spectrum of possible interpretations to the opposite end, it may seem that the principle of equal access is consistent with rather little medical care being provided. As long as there is equal access to whatever modest level of care is supplied, the principle may seem to be satisfied. But that is not plausible, because part of the case for insisting that access to medical care should be equal is surely the conviction that medical care is very important, and supplying rather little of it is then scarcely consistent with that conviction.

A satisfactory formulation of the equal access principle is going to reside somewhere in the considerable space between the opposite ends of the spectrum explored above. I am going to examine two distinct lines of thought that converge upon, or at least are consistent with, the same formulation.

An argument from insurance

Our problem is to determine the amount of health care to which there should be equal access. This problem is encompassed by the notionally larger question of determining the amount of health care that should be provided. One way of approaching this latter question and giving it a more concrete form is by posing it within an insurance-based system, in which individuals determine for themselves how much health care it is sensible to provide. The answer will crucially depend upon the resources at their disposal. Let us therefore suppose, at least, that individuals are given a fair allocation of goods, however that is to be construed, prior to making their insurance decisions, for that seems a precondition of the resultant distribution of health care being morally acceptable. What level of cover will it be rational for individuals to take out?

Though the circumstances are very abstractly described, certain conclusions nevertheless emerge. It will not seem rational for someone to take out no cover, since that will expose him or her to the real risk of being unable to afford vital but expensive treatment for very serious illness. With cover, the cost will be spread amongst the insured group and become affordable. Conversely, some levels and forms of cover will seem excessive because they divert too many resources from other important undertakings in his or her life. Furthermore if the fair allocation of goods referred to above involves an unequal distribution of goods, then it is likely to be rational for people to take out different levels of health insurance. Having spent a certain amount on health cover, less well off people may not find it rational to spend more, given other demands on their money, whereas better-off individuals with more funds to meet those other demands may find it rational to spend some of their surplus on further health cover.

These conclusions may be not merely about the amount of health care it is rational to provide, but also about the distribution of health care it is just to provide. There is a tradition of supposing that a distribution of goods determined by the rational prudence of individuals choosing in an initially fair situation is at once a just distribution of goods.[7] This is not the place to explore the merits of that conception of justice, but we can at least ask the pertinent question whether it can really be an obligation of justice on the rest of us to supply an individual with a level of health care for which he would not have found it rational to insure himself. If it cannot be, then these conclusions about the rationality of different levels of health cover do have a bearing on what justice requires with respect to health care.

What then is this bearing, in particular with respect to the question of equal access? Must there be equal access to equal health care? Since it seems likely to be rational for people to take out the same level of health care insurance only if they have equal wealth initially, this suggests that justice requires access to equal health care provision only if it also requires more general economic equality. This is an important conclusion because it contradicts the rather common view that, even though economic inequality is permissible, health care, being special, requires to be distributed equally. If indeed justice does not demand full economic equality, as many will think, and so equal access to equal health care is not required, what is required on this view? Even though people of different means will rationally insure themselves for different levels of health care, there is a level of provision that all will find it rational to make. The natural inference to draw is that what there should be equal access to is this level of health care. We may think of this as a particular interpretation of the familiar idea that there should be equal access to a decent minimum of health care, where the decent minimum is construed as that level of health care which it is rational for everyone to insure for, given a fair allocation of resources.

In the line of thought just unfolded the questions have been posed from, and the answers reflect, the point of view of the insurant. These answers will be suspect to those who suppose that the perspective of the patient will have to figure, more prominently than it does in the above argument, in a credible account of a just distribution of health care. Even if it is not rational for the person *qua* insurant to cover himself for a certain treatment, that same person *qua* patient, if such he becomes, will need the treatment, and that may be thought to ground a just claim on his part to the treatment. This observation initiates the second of the two lines of thought that I wish to pursue in an effort to arrive at a satisfactory formulation of the equal access principle.

An argument from equal opportunity

One of the more widely shared principles of justice in our society is that of equality of opportunity. The ideal is, very broadly, that the range of opportunities provided by our culture should be equally accessible to all. The breadth of support for this principle is no doubt facilitated by its inherent vagueness, but it provides a starting point for thinking about health care. For there is no opportunity that cannot be extinguished by one sort of ill health or another, and so the provision of health care is one of the most fundamental things that needs to be done to secure equality of opportunity.[8] A principle of equal opportunity effectively amounts to a principle of equal access, and, as we have seen, underlying that ideal is a metaphysical vision of human beings as autonomous choosers and an allied morality of respect for choice. Once again autonomy is vulnerable to ill health and so its maintenance requires the provision of health care. Thus the principle of equal opportunity and its underlying value of autonomy converge in requiring that health care needs should be met, and met equally, presumably. What are the implications of this line of argument for the amount of health care that must be supplied and to which there must be equal access?

Health care that is necessary to secure equal opportunity and to protect autonomy will be morally required, and this is clearly going to incorporate an extensive repertoire of fundamental treatments designed to save life, cure disease and overcome disability.

174

But equally evidently there are many lesser forms of health care whose impact upon opportunity and autonomy seems likely to be negligible and whose provision therefore would not be required by justice. Moreover in determining the quantity of provision it is to be remembered that it is health need and care that we are discussing, because there are forms of intervention delivered in a conventional medical setting which are only misleadingly thought of as health care. Let us compare abortion and infertility treatment in this respect.

In discussions of whether or not the latter should be provided on the NHS, it is sometimes said that it should not be, because it is not really medical treatment in so far as it is not designed to cure a disease. While infertility may be the consequence of a disease, it is not itself a disease. But this is implausible, because in so far as medicine is credibly understood as aiming to restore normal biological function to a patient, it encompasses the correcting of disability as well as the curing of disease, and infertility, if not a disease, is certainly a disability. It may be countered, however, that infertility treatment does not correct the disability, but only outflanks it. The patient remains infertile in the natural sense, but is enabled to have a child by ingenious medical technology. But that in its turn is unsatisfactory, for if health care is allowed to cover the restoration of physical ability to a person, it seems reasonable to construe it as extending to cover the provision of a functional equivalent to the ability, if the ability cannot itself be restored. Thus the provision of artificial devices to enable a person to walk or to see seems credibly to fall within the ambit of health care, and so should infertility treatment, which provides a functional equivalent of natural fertility.

By contrast abortion, leaving aside the genuinely therapeutic cases, is not a matter of health care. Being with child is neither a disease nor a disability and termination of the pregnancy is not grounded in a health care need. The need, if need it is, is social, despite spurious attempts to inflate the therapeutic to encompass the social. On this account, then, the argument of justice that requires the provision of certain health care services does not apply to abortion, though it does to the provision of infertility services, since infertility, unlike pregnancy, constitutes a health care need and moreover thwarts an important human opportunity, namely to have a family.

This is an important conclusion, since it suggests that the distribution of current opinion is the wrong way round, with few challenging the provision of abortion on the NHS aside from those who regard abortion as wrong, and rather more opposing the provision of infertility services. This is not to say that there may not be other possible lines of argument for the provision of abortion services, perhaps even to do with equal opportunity and autonomy, since the availability of abortion has been argued to be necessary if women are to control their bodies. But it is a further task to develop such lines of argument satisfactorily, and it remains important to see that the case for the provision of abortion services is not simply an aspect of the general requirement of justice to provide a certain level of health care.

This second line of argument for determining the content of the equal access principle thus yields the conclusion that there should be equal access to a central core of health care that helps to sustain equal opportunity and autonomy, but not necessarily to care that has no impact on these things, nor to care that is not truly health care. As with the first line of argument, we may construe this upshot as a particular interpretation of the idea that there should be equal access to a decent minimum of health care. What that decent minimum should contain on this interpretation will not be capable of precise determination. Different medical procedures will make varying contributions to maintaining equality of opportunity and autonomy, from the considerable to the negligible, and it will be a matter of judgement whether the contribution made by a particular procedure is in all the circumstances, including other calls on resources, sufficient to warrant its inclusion in the decent minimum.

Arguably that judgement is best arrived at through the political process. Philosophy may be able to offer some guidance as to the parameters of an acceptable allocation of health care, but politics is better suited to determine it more precisely. Placing the decision in the hands of the voter may seem to bring this line of argument closer to the first one. In the latter the insurant has to determine how much of his resources to devote to health insurance, and now in the present line of argument the voter has to determine what counts as a decent minimum. The worry, referred to above, that the perspective of the sick is not adequately accommodated in the first line of argument seems applicable to this line of argument too. But in both cases the worry is misplaced. The insurant has to balance the interest he has as a potentially healthy person in not spending too much on insurance against the interest he has as a potentially sick person in spending rather more. Similarly the voter must balance the interests of the sick and the healthy in determining what is a decent minimum of health care. The perspective of the sick is accommodated in both cases without being the sole perspective in either.

WEALE, CAVERS AND SELF-RESPECT

The fact that two rather different ways of thinking about the allocation of health care converge upon, or are at least consistent with, an interpretation of the equal access principle in terms of a decent minimum lends weight to that interpretation. Albert Weale's formulation of the principle is rather different, to the effect that 'comprehensive, high-quality medical care should be available to all citizens on test of professionally judged medical need and without financial barriers to access'.[9] In other words, there should be equal access to comprehensive, high-quality medical care. Weale wonders whether this version of the principle constitutes an inconsistent triad of propositions, in the current circumstances of rising medical costs and a declining disposition to tolerate high social expenditure. Perhaps in these circumstances comprehensiveness, high quality and access to all are not simultaneously achievable, though any two of them may be. With respect to each element he explores the case for dropping it while retaining the other two. He concludes that we cannot credibly abandon any of the elements entirely, but must accept and negotiate, presumably by compromise, the conflict of values embedded in the principle, just as we accept and negotiate conflicts of value elsewhere in public policy.

On the version of the equal access principle that I have promoted, two and perhaps all three of Weale's elements are compromised. What there is to be access to is not comprehensive medical care but only a decent minimum, and while that minimum should be of good quality it may not be of the highest. When it comes to equality of access, there is equal access to the decent minimum but not necessarily to anything beyond it. The availability of anything further is going to depend upon one's personal resources. The practical implications of his position and mine may not be very different, but the attitude towards them would be. What Weale would presumably regard as compromises of justice forced by scarcity I would regard as consistent with the best interpretation of the equal access principle.

177

Weale, I take it, supposes that the NHS complies, more or less, with his version of the equal access principle. By contrast David Cavers seems to think it is more in line with the decent minimum version of the principle, or even something less. Thus he describes the NHS as a 'safety net only . . . working to a lowest common denominator in health care provision'.[10] This language suggests something rather less acceptable than a decent minimum, and Cavers thinks that more money needs to be got into health care. But, given the state of contemporary political opinion, he judges that there is no serious chance of the money being forthcoming from public funds, leaving private provision as the only source. In his view it is not just necessary for it to come from this source but also desirable, and he looks forward to what he calls a mixed economy of health care, combining public and private provision. The private sector needs to be, and can be made, much more competitive and less expensive than it is at present, thus attracting much more money than it does at present. Those who take out private insurance will still be contributing towards the NHS but not, so to speak, drawing on that contribution, thereby leaving more resources in the system for others. Everybody will apparently gain.

The primary moral objection that may be made to these proposals is that they infringe the principle of equal access, because access to private provision will depend upon one's resources. But if my account of that principle is correct, this objection fails. If NHS provision under Cavers's arrangements meets the standard of a decent minimum, then, since there is equal access to the NHS, there is equal access to what the principle requires. That access to private provision above the minimum is not equal is no infringement of the principle.

Cavers is anxious to encourage more private provision in health care, and one feature of the present arrangements that may be thought to discourage it is the fact that those who make it receive no relief from their contribution to the NHS. Despite this Cavers shows no disposition to alter this arrangement, because to do so would lead to a complete break between private and public provision 'that might have serious overtones of social division'.[11] There may be various reasons for being concerned about social division, but one is that it may undermine the self-respect of those on the less advantaged side of the division. Indeed, Cavers's own proposals, though they offer private insurants no relief from NHS contributions, may still be charged with injuring self-respect in so far as they allow, and indeed encourage, the better-off to obtain more of something as valuable as health care. This is, of course, a challenge not merely to Cavers's proposals, but also to the decent minimum interpretation of the equal access principle that they seem to embody and that I have defended.

Is, then, the self-respect of those who receive only the decent minimum of health care likely to be injured? There is no reason why it should be if the two alternative arguments for the decent minimum interpretation of the equal access principle are recalled. Why, to invoke the first argument, should a person's self-respect be injured by receipt of a decent minimum if he would have had no reason to provide more than that for himself had he been left to make his own insurance arrangements? Why, to invoke the second argument, should a person's self-respect be undermined by receipt of a decent minimum if that minimum is sufficient to ensure equal opportunity and an autonomous life, both of which seem central to the maintenance of self-respect? But, it may be said in reply, whether or not the provision of a decent minimum of health care coupled with the freedom to buy more should rationally injure self-respect, the fact is that in practice it is likely to do so in our society, with its post-war tradition of access to more or less equal health care. It is true, of course, that during that period people have continued to take out private insurance, but the NHS has not been conceived of as only a decent minimum, and its apparent philosophy of access to equal care has done much to enhance the self-respect of citizens. This, it may be said, would be undermined by an overt reinterpretation of the NHS as a decent minimum and an encouragement of much more widespread and extensive private provision.

There is perhaps some truth in this argument, but the grounds of self-respect are not immutable. In different societies it may be fostered by different things. It may be that in Britain, which has perhaps more considerable economic and social inequalities than most other Western societies, our health care arrangements have come to bear a peculiar burden of sustaining self-respect. But, if that is true, the conclusion to be drawn from it is not that those arrangements should be regarded as sacrosanct, even though there are other good reasons for altering them, but rather that the burden of sustaining self-respect should be partially redistributed to other social arrangements. Thus a diminution in social and economic inequalities would foster people's self-respect, thereby diminishing the burden borne by health care to achieve the same end. Our moral understanding of health care could then be reconceived in terms of entitlement to a decent minimum without undue harm to the springs of self-respect, particularly if emphasis was placed upon the reasons why such a reconception rationally constitutes no insult to those who receive the decent minimum.

NOTES

1 Page 138.
2 Ibid.
3 David Cavers, Chapter 8, pp. 151–164, of this volume.
4 Ibid.
5 Ibid.
6 Onora O'Neill, 'Opportunities, equalities and education', *Theory and Decision* 7 (1976), pp. 275–95.
7 For this general conception of justice see John Rawls, *A Theory of Justice*, Clarendon Press, Oxford, 1972. For its application in the domain of health care, with respect to age, see Norman Daniels, *Am I my Parents' Keeper?*, Oxford University Press, Oxford, 1988.
8 Norman Daniels, 'Health-care needs and distributive justice', *Philosophy and Public Affairs* 10, 2 (1981), 146–79.
9 Chapter 7 above, p. 139.
10 Chapter 8, p. 152.
11 Ibid., p. 158.

10

PUBLIC OR PRIVATE?

Insurance and pensions

P. M. Booth and G. M. Dickinson

THE PROBLEMS OF STATE INSURANCE PROVISION

The state does provide, only the state can provide?

One of the strongest arguments against the private provision of insurance which is currently provided by the state is that, without it, millions of people would be uninsured and receive sub-standard services as, it is alleged, happened before the 1948 National Assistance Act. This argument is flawed. It is based on a misreading of history. Before the Second World War, millions of people, even on quite modest incomes, obtained insurance benefits from friendly societies, other types of insurers, unions and voluntary organisations: see, for example, Seldon *et al.* (1996). However, to compare insurance provision before the war with state provision now is not to compare like with like. The quality and variety of all goods and services have improved since the war beyond all measure. If the state had nationalised the production of refrigerators, some advance in technology and market coverage might have occurred since the war; people might then have argued that it had happened because of the control of production by the state. In fact, we all know that the product has improved beyond all measure because the state has *not* been involved in its production. We should not assume that, because the state has provided social insurance, and because the quality and coverage in some areas have increased, that they have increased because of the role of the state rather than despite the role of the state.

Choice and efficiency

Thus, if the public can be persuaded that a private market in the provision of social insurance is possible, what are its benefits? Currently, much social insurance derives from a compulsory contract between the state and the individual. If that contract were not enforced, many individuals might gain from not taking out a particular insurance or from taking it out in a different form. In a private market, people would face prices which would reflect the actual cost of the insurance. They could then choose how they wished to spend their own money; choose the quantity and type of insurance they wished to purchase; choose whether they wished to be uninsured or whether they wished to change their behaviour in a way which made insurance less necessary. Numerous examples could be given to illustrate how a private market can satisfy individual needs better. We will restrict ourselves to a few examples. Much is made of the costs of the US health care system, particularly of the costs of litigation. However, the positive points are rarely mentioned. Seldon (1981) shows how the number of doctors per patient in the US has outstripped that in the UK and has risen much faster as incomes have risen. In the UK the proportion of income spent on health insurance is stuck at the politically ideal proportion. Health is an income-elastic product. In the politicised UK system, people cannot spend more as income rises, unless they pay twice for a whole range of services by using and paying for both private and state care.

As well as restricting the amount people spend, state-provided insurance imposes a uniform contract and service. It is feasible, in a private market, for people to purchase different packages of health and other insurances. One package could have a longer waiting time for operations but more provision for labour-intensive geriatric care. Another package might provide better 'hotel facilities'. In the field of long-term care a whole range of products and methods of financing care (annual premiums, immediate needs annuities, house sale, etc.) can be used to suit the needs of the individual. In a tax-financed social insurance system, there is one product, one price and one level of cover. A similar situation exists with unemployment insurance. Two important variables which affect the risk and the degree of moral hazard and which would therefore affect the premium quite dramatically are the waiting period (the time before any benefit is paid) and the maximum benefit payment period. Individuals with substantial savings may want a long waiting period. Mobile individuals who work in industries where work can be seasonal may want a short waiting period with a relatively short maximum payment period. With state unemployment benefit, there is normally one price, one benefit level, one waiting period and one maximum benefit period. Private markets would also be more innovative than the state in terms of the methods used to provide consumers with income protection. Whilst a uniform state benefit may have been satisfactory at times when economies were stable, it is clearly not appropriate in today's changing world. Different people in different professions and at different ages will have different work patterns and different social insurance needs. One of the great virtues of the market is producers' ability to respond to price signals and the profit motive to innovate and develop products to meet consumers' needs in ways which could not be envisaged by those controlling state-provided insurance. Friendly societies, with-profit policies and unit-linked contracts are just three examples of how private markets have developed products to meet different consumer needs for risk protection. Private long-term care insurers have also proved to be more successful than local authorities in finding methods to care for people in their own home rather than moving them into a residential care home.

Moral hazard

Individuals may have different behavioural preferences when they are not faced with the true economic costs of their behaviour. Perhaps the most obvious example is health insurance. If private renewable-annual-premium health insurance were widely marketed, doubtless, there would be differential premiums for smokers and non-smokers. Smokers would face the true cost of their behaviour in terms of higher health insurance premiums. They might choose to modify their behaviour rather than pay higher premiums. There is a political danger, in fact, of not allowing people to face the full cost of their social behavioural decisions. It was one of the main arguments in Hayek's *Road to Serfdom* that government interference in the economic field gradually led to greater interference in the political and social field and the building up of more and more bureaucracy and arbitrary powers. The reason for this is clear in health. People's lifestyle decisions are a most important determinant of their health. When the government is paying for health care, it may begin to take a greater interest in people's life style. This has happened to quite a large extent in the UK and in the late 1990s, with a more interventionist Labour government, one can see the trend developing. The previous government's *Health of the Nation* document was clearly an attempt to influence people's life styles. The EU-wide restrictions on tobacco advertising and sponsorship are another example. There is more and more legislation in the safety field as well as much money spent by quangos on influencing life style. Legislation such as that promoting compulsory seat belts is often justified, not on paternalistic grounds, but on the financial grounds of the benefit to the NHS.

It is clear that our social insurance system has significant incentives towards moral hazard. Moral hazard is not absent in private insurance markets but there are effective ways of dealing with it. Some of these will be discussed below. However, at the most basic level, policy deductibles, waiting periods and the more effective scrutinising of claims all help to reduce moral hazard. Such mechanisms are much more difficult to develop for state-provided insurance because of the requirement for uniform policy conditions and because of the desire to achieve complete coverage of the population. Thus, for example, although the state uses various mechanisms to scrutinise the legitimacy of claims for unemployment benefit, it is very difficult to prevent somebody who is unwilling to work from claiming some state benefits, even if those benefits are social security benefits rather than unemployment benefit. Whilst part of the increase in social security budgets in recent years relates to the increase in the number of old people, and some may be due to an apparent decrease in the demand for unskilled labour, much of the increase must have arisen as a result of a gradual change in behaviour by people who, being insured by the state, are not deterred from adopting a particular life style by the financial consequences.

Policy-induced risk

Lindbeck (1994) suggests that the problem of controlling moral hazard leads the government constantly to change the rules regarding the availability of state-provided insurances, thus creating 'policy-induced risk'. This is a further major disadvantage of state-provided insurances. If the state is unable to control moral hazard except by changing policy conditions, people will be uncertain as to the extent to which they are covered by a state-provided insurance or, indeed, as to whether they are covered at all. The changing of the disability benefit rules in the UK (and its replacement by incapacity benefit) is one example of policy-induced risk arising due to the state being unable to control moral hazard. Another manifestation of policy-induced risk is the way governments can crowd out private insurance by providing state benefits and then suddenly withdraw from provision, leaving a situation where people cannot get protection from the state and where the private market is not sufficiently well developed for people to buy private insurance. A recent example of this problem was seen in the UK with the reduction in the state's support for mortgage interest, leaving people to insure privately, in a market which had been prevented from developing by the existence of state-provided benefits. Some would argue that a similar situation was evident in health care.

Policy-induced risk is an inherent problem with state-provided insurance, and very little can be done to reduce it. Indeed, as social insurance systems become an increasing burden on the taxpayer as the working population ages, this problem may be exacerbated. There are two inherent problems with state insurances which can make them far more risky than private insurances. First, there is no enforceable contract. One of the purposes of the state is to develop law and procedures of justice which ensure that private contracts are enforced. Yet the state, unless it enters into explicit contracts, which it does very rarely, can withdraw or change a benefit at any time it wishes. Whether an insurance benefit is paid will depend on the wishes of voters at the time a benefit is due, expressed through the democratic system. Voters may renege on promises made by previous groups of voters because they may become unaffordable or because voters have other political priorities.

A related problem is that the democratic mechanism, through which state insurance is controlled, can develop inherent conflicts between groups in society. Different groups can use the democratic system to achieve economic aims for which they do not meet the cost. Those aims can be achieved only by thwarting the aims of others (for example, by reducing their income by extra taxation). When others in the system see that they are economically disadvantaged by this, they may then withdraw, through the democratic system, the economic privileges which have been granted to another group. This is clearly happening with social insurance schemes in continental Europe. A free market resolves such conflicts by ensuring that every individual who enters a contract is responsible for the costs of his activities. A private contract which is negotiated in a free market is freely entered by both parties and must be beneficial to both parties. Of course, there are different risks in a private insurance market; some of these, such as the risk of insurer insolvency, can be reduced by certain types of regulation. Those risks can also be reduced by competition. When insurance is provided by the state, there is only one provider. The customer has no way of controlling the policy risk. If a government, under the cloak of democratic legitimacy, decides to reduce the pension benefits to a particular generation, nothing can be done to mitigate those risks by the citizens affected.

These problems do not mean, of course, that income should not be redistributed through the political system. Although the extensive social insurance and pensions systems in continental Europe have become politically and economically unsustainable, there is clearly political support for providing a basic income and income supplements for both the old and the working generations.

Dynamic efficiency

The authors also believe that insurance services would be produced more efficiently if they were produced in private markets. It is our general experience that privatisation of state industries and services has brought enormous benefits in terms of efficiency and production. However, efficiency should not be seen just in static terms. It is often said that the state provides some insurance benefits at a lower unit administrative cost than the private sector would be able to provide them. Indeed, Booth and Stroinski (1996) make that point in the discussion of the Polish social insurance system. However, whilst it may be true that, at a given time, the state could nationalise a system, make it universal, impose the same benefit scales on everybody and then administer the system more cheaply than the private sector, this is not to compare like with like. First, a private system is likely to develop a more diverse range of insurance products which may appear to cost more to administer but add value because they can be adapted to suit individual need. Second, a state system which may start administratively efficient would gradually become bureaucratic, inefficient and less responsive to the customer. Third, part of a private insurer's expenditure will be on claims control; the state may appear to be more efficient in this regard but simply suffers from a higher level of fraudulent claims (there is well documented evidence of this in the Polish pension system amongst disability claimants, also discussed in Booth and Stroinski (1996)).

UNSUSTAINABLE SOLIDARITY
BETWEEN THE GENERATIONS

In this section, we focus on the problems caused by unfunded social insurance schemes providing long-term benefits. We will see that many of the benefits provided in social insurance schemes are only partly insurance benefits. To a large extent they are benefits that the private sector would often provide through savings rather than insurance. This leads to a whole new set of problems from state-provided social insurance which are of a particularly acute nature in the EU.

Funded and Paygo

When we consider pensions and other benefits which normally require an element of saving, we can divide the mechanisms of providing such benefits into funded and pay-as-you-go provision. When we talk about funded insurance benefits, we are referring to the mechanism of provision whereby money is set aside and invested in order to meet future contingencies. Unfunded, or pay-as-you-go, benefits are met not from capital accumulation and saving but from the taxes of the working generation.

Different systems give rise to different risks. A funded system gives rise to the risk that investments may not be successful and may not give rise to a sufficiently high return to meet benefits. However, the mechanism of funding gives rise to a control mechanism whereby an appraisal of the scheme or a valuation can be performed every year and an adjustment made to the contribution rate to the scheme if investments are underperforming expectations.

With unfunded or pay-as-you-go systems, the cost of one generation's pensions is met from the taxes of the working generation. The main risk here is that the demographic profile of the population will change, so that there will be insufficient workers in a given generation to meet the payments to the retired generation. This will happen if the population ages through either a fall in death rates or a reduction in birth rates. The problem of unfunded schemes is illustrated by the current demographic situation in Europe. After the war there was an increase in the birth rate followed by a sharp fall in the birth rate and a fall in mortality rates. In the unfunded arrangements, the large post-war working generation paid relatively low taxes or social insurance contributions to pay the pensions of the small pensioner generation. When this large working generation is retired and living longer, the smaller generation behind will have to pay very high taxes to meet the cost of the pensions. There is an implicit debt building up in the system because the large working generation are building up a pension entitlement which they are not financing. The size and nature of that debt will be discussed below.

These difficulties with unfunded insurance benefits arise whenever there is a long-term savings element to an insurance benefit. Thus, for example, health insurance, long-term care, pensions and whole-life and widows' benefits should all involve a significant element of saving, in that capital should be put aside today to meet the benefits to be paid in the future, which cannot be met from current income, at a later stage in life.

Arguments have been put forward, for example by Brown (1995), which suggest that there is macro-economic equivalence between funded and unfunded arrangements. The argument was effectively articulated by the editor of the professional magazine *The Actuary*. There it was suggested that whether benefits are funded or not is irrelevant because all must consume what the workers produce in aggregate, whether or not benefits are funded. Therefore the pensions of today's pensioners must come from the product of today's workers. This argument is a fallacy (as was pointed out in correspondence by Arthur, Booth and Green in *The Actuary*, 1996). The argument is based on the error of aggregation so common in Keynesian economics. By concentrating on aggregate concepts, the whole point of funding is missed. Individuals partake in capital investment which can raise the productivity of the next generation and thereby provide the means to pay their pensions without additional effort on behalf of workers. It also ignores the fact that funded schemes permit international investment, which allows countries with an ageing population to obtain equity stakes in the emerging economies of the world, which tend to have younger populations.

Europe's demographic problems

Kessler (1996) discusses the demographic problems which have led to pressures on social insurance systems and proposes different ways of preventing intergenerational conflicts. We discuss some of those issues here. There has been a fall in fertility and a rise in life expectancy in nearly all developed countries, shown in Table 10.1. The impact of these demographic changes will be felt over the next fifty years. The old age dependence ratio is forecast by the United

Table 10.1 Fertility and life expectancy in EU countries, 1950 *v.* 1990

Country	Fertility rate (children per woman)		Life expectancy (years)	
	1950	1990	1950	1990
France	2.9	1.8	62.9	72.8
Netherlands	3.1	1.6	70.6	73.8
UK	2.2	1.8	66.2	72.0

Source: de la Fuente (1995); Taverne (1995).

Nations, reported in Besseling and Zeeuw (1993), to increase, over the EU as a whole, from 19.3 in 1970 to 39.9 in 2050. One of the most dramatic increases is forecast in Italy, where it is forecast to increase from 16.9 to 45.7.

Meeting Paygo liabilities: the magnitude of the problem

The financial unsustainability of pay-as-you-go state pension schemes can be illustrated in a number of ways. First, we could look at the level of contributions that will have to be paid in future years if the benefits promised by the state are to be met. Second, we could look at long-term budget deficits and national debt figures for countries on the assumption that their state social insurance schemes remain intact. Third, we could calculate the 'actuarial value'[1] of the benefits promised to future generations which have not been funded. Whichever method is used provides some alarming statistics. Taking the first approach to quantifying the financial burden of future pension liabilities, Besseling and Zeeuw (1993) find that, without reform, average EU contribution rates to finance state benefits would have to increase from a level of 15.2 per cent of gross wages in 1990 to 23.2 per cent of gross wages in 2030. These figures exclude other social insurance benefits paid to the elderly and, of course, will disguise variations within the average figure. Chand and Jaeger (1996), writing for the IMF, estimate the sustainable contribution rate which it would be necessary to charge, over a long period, to prevent the system getting any more in debt. This is shown, for a number of countries, in Table 10.2. It should be noted that, if this rate were charged, it would not extinguish any of the existing debt and, if the sustainable rate were not immediately introduced from the base date of the

Table 10.2 Increases in sustainable contribution rates

Country	% of GDP
Germany	3.4
France	3.3
Italy	2.5
UK	0.1

Source: Chand and Jaeger (1996).

projection, 1995, the contribution rates would have to increase much further in future years.

The figures in Table 10.2 are percentages of GDP and imply a higher increase in social security taxes which are not paid on the whole of national income. If countries do not set a sustainable contribution rate which can meet pension liabilities over the long term, it will be necessary for them to adjust social security taxes on a year-to-year basis to meet pay-as-you-go liabilities as they accrue. The numbers then appear more dramatic. At the extremes, Italy would eventually require a contribution rate of 68.2 per cent of its wage bill and the UK 5 per cent of its wage bill.

The OECD (reported in Paribas, 1995) has taken the second approach to measuring the cost of all social insurance benefits. The projections assume that all policy changes announced at the time were undertaken. Germany was projected to have a budget deficit of 9 per cent of GDP by 2030, with a debt to GDP ratio of over 100 per cent. The figures for France are similar. Italy was projected to have a budget deficit of 13 per cent by 2030 and a debt to GDP ratio of 120 per cent (that assumes that ambitious budget cuts under discussion actually took place). The UK, with its low state pay-as-you-go and high level of funded pensions, has a projected budget surplus and a projected debt to GDP ratio of below 10 per cent.

When looking at the actuarial value of benefits which have not been funded, we can take two approaches. First, we can look at the total value of all liabilities which have been promised to those currently working or receiving pensions: this is the total unfunded burden and would be the cost that would have to be met by current contributors if there were an immediate switch to funded provision but with the state still meeting existing commitments. Second, we can look at the smaller figure of the difference between the actuarial value of benefits and actuarial value of contributions if they are paid

190

Table 10.3 Net pension liability (after allowing for future contributions)

Country	% of GDP
UK	4.6
Germany	110.7
France	113.6
Italy	75.5

Source: Chand and Jaeger (1996).

at their current rate. The distinction between these two debts is important in policy terms and is considered in greater detail below. Just considering the second part of the debt (the lower figure) we still get some disturbing results, shown in Table 10.3.

A more detailed assessment of EU pension liabilities can be found in Franco and Munzi (1996), although the figures produced in that report, for different countries, cannot be compared with each other directly.

There are two reasons why different countries have different unfunded pension burdens. One of these relates to the different extent to which demographic difficulties have developed in different countries. The other relates to the balance between private and state provision. We would expect that those countries which have the greatest private provision would have the most developed long-term institutional investment markets. This is certainly true. As a percentage of GDP, UK pension fund assets are 79 per cent, German pension fund assets 6 per cent, French pension fund assets 3 per cent and Italian pension fund assets 1 per cent. (It is worth noting that the Netherlands has pension fund assets greater than the UK in GDP terms.) These issues are discussed in De Ryck (1996). It is also of interest to note that UK pension funds tend to own a greater proportion of the listed equities in the UK and that a greater proportion of assets tends to be invested in equities and other private sector investments.

Social solidarity or political conflict and social insecurity?

Thus the benefits promised under state pay-as you-go social insurance schemes are benefits which have to be met, not by the returns from a large pool of savings and investments, but from future taxes. One of the challenges of this chapter is to demonstrate how these financial liabilities can be unwound whilst meeting, as closely as possible, the aspirations of those who were promised benefits by politicians who knew that it would be their successors who would have to pay the costs of their promises.

However, we should look deeper into the problem of social insurance liabilities than the mere financial costs. There are worrying social implications of setting up systems for which the individual is not responsible. One principle of free-market economics is that a system can be relatively controlled if those who take a particular action face all the costs and benefits of that action. With pay-as-you-go pension schemes taxpayers as a whole, from a given working generation, pay the pensions, as a whole, of the retired generation. There is no self-correcting mechanism which ensures stability. There is no incentive, for example, for an individual to have sufficient children, simply to ensure that pay-as-you-go pensions can be financed. In a pay-as-you-go collective pension scheme, transfers are socialised so that there is no incentive within the system for any individual to take action that can sustain the system. The only way the system can be sustained would be if policy decisions were taken by governments to force people to have larger families, to encourage immigration or to reduce the elderly population (for example, taking decisions regarding euthanasia not on the grounds of the ethical and philosophical arguments but on the grounds of the cost to the state of keeping the elderly population). This is a further manifestation of the observation of Hayek (1945) that increasing control of decisions by government in the social and political sphere can arise as a result of control of economic decisions. Thus there is a philosophical problem that the socialisation of pay-as-you-go pension schemes could undermine basic political freedoms because the government is financially responsible for the fertility patterns of individuals and therefore may wish to influence social decisions.

The provision of generous social insurance benefits is often described as providing 'solidarity between the generations'; it is often justified according to the so-called principles of social justice. This description and justification are meaningless and dangerous. The process of promising benefits to the aged, in a system which is not funded, involves one generation, through the ballot box, voting for pension promises which are to be funded by a generation which may not yet even vote and may, indeed, not yet even be born. It is difficult to conceive of a policy which is more likely to lead to conflict between generations, particularly if, as we have noted, the generation which has promised itself insurance benefits does not produce the children who are needed to pay the taxes to finance those benefits. It is also difficult to envisage a system which could be as unjust as voting pension costs on to successive generations without providing them with the means to meet those costs.

The possible nature of future conflict between the generations is described in Kessler (1996). What will happen if today's young people decide that they do not wish their standard of living to fall as a result of the pension promises which have been made to future generations? Will they express their dissatisfaction by non-political means? If one appreciates that the growing elderly population will form a greater proportion of the electorate, will the government be able to take that action which is necessary to move towards sustainable systems of funding which will create genuine solidarity between generations?

One reason why some people prefer state-provided benefits to privately funded benefits is that they perceive that there is less risk attached to benefits provided by the state. This feeling is likely to be more prominent where the state has been more or less the only provider of insurance-type benefits. Skrabski (1996) found that faith in state-provided pension benefits was much greater than faith in voluntary provision in Hungary. In the UK it is likely that the general public would have more confidence in state-provided health care than in privately provided health care. However, a different result might be found in an area where private provision had not been crowded out by state provision, such as pensions (although there does appear to be a willingness to continue to pay basic levels of pension). But it is a mistake to think that, under all circumstances, the state can be a guarantor of adequate benefits. Lindbeck (1994) discusses the problem of *policy-induced risk*. This can take three forms. First, the political system may not be able to deliver benefits which were promised by previous generations of politicians. Second, voter preferences may change so that benefits paid under social security rules are reduced. Third, the government may be obliged to keep changing the rules to prevent loopholes and abuses developing. Under these circumstances, social *in*security replaces social security because intergenerational transfers made through the state are not enforceable, in the same way that a private contract is enforceable. Social conflict may then replace social solidarity.

CAN PRIVATE INSURANCE DELIVER?

Let us look at the issue of the extent to which the private sector could in principle supply insurance contracts in those areas now provided by social security systems. Before looking at this, it is useful to recap on the preconditions which need to exist for the provision of private insurance to take place. There are four main preconditions.

- First, insurance companies must have sufficient information to allow them to price the risks against which they offer protection. Information must be sufficient not just to ensure that the overall level of premiums charged is sufficient to meet the expected claims paid and associated administration and capital support costs. It is also necessary that the information is adequate to allow discriminatory pricing. Discriminatory pricing here means that the price charged relates to the expected cost. This can be viewed as 'fair' pricing from the standpoint of the consumer. In a competitive insurance market, discriminatory pricing is necessary if there is to be an adequate and sustainable supply.
- Second, in a voluntary market anti-selection must be kept within tolerable levels, either by efficient screening (e.g. medical tests in the field of disability insurance and health insurance, etc.) or the insurance companies must be able to forecast the level of anti-selection and build it into the premiums they charge without causing the 'fair pricing' system to be significantly undermined.
- Third, moral hazard must be capable of being kept within tolerable levels, e.g. through contract design (e.g. deductibles, waiting periods before claims are paid, etc.) or through incentives (e.g. no-claim discounts) in the pricing mechanism.
- Fourth, the risk concentrations facing the insurance company must not be too great. Large-scale losses, such as those caused by natural catastrophes, stretch the risk absorption capacity of the insurance industry. Significant levels of correlation between smaller individual risk exposures due to an underlying common economic cause (e.g. collapse of the property market) can similarly give rise to loss concentration. The capacity of private insurance companies to accept loss concentration is reasonably high, since they have an efficient system for sharing large potential losses globally through reinsurance. When there are risk concentrations through major catastrophes or through correlations across a portfolio of individual risks, the cost of insurance

will necessarily be higher, because the law of large numbers does not apply as effectively.

Hence, when looking at whether private insurance markets could replace social security provision, it is important to keep these four preconditions in mind.

The main areas of social security provision can be grouped into four main areas: retirement provision, health care financing (including long-term care), unemployment insurance and disability insurances. In addition, there are a range of financial supports to cover family-related adversities, such as breakdown of marriage, maternity costs, etc. One can group all these various protections offered under social security systems into two main categories:

- The maintenance of a threshold level of income over time, e.g. pensions allow the maintenance of income in the state of retirement, long-term disability insurances allow maintenance of income during sickness or accident, and, of course, unemployment insurance defines itself.
- Financial support to cover major additional expenditures arising from adverse 'life events', e.g. hospitalisation, bodily impairment, etc. Indeed, this support for major additional expenditures can also be viewed as part of the maintenance of a threshold level of *disposable* income (where 'disposable' income is used in a wider sense than the conventional economic sense) over time.

Let us look at the issue of the extent to which private sector insurance could in principle replace state provision in these areas. We shall exclude here the family-related protections, such as family breakdown, maternity costs, etc.

Retirement provision

It goes without saying that pension provision is a well established area of supply for life insurance companies and for other private sector suppliers. Let us apply the four preconditions of insurability discussed above. In the first place, information for the insurance pricing component of pensions is concerned essentially with having adequate mortality tables to forecast longevity. Actuarial tables are well developed and hence this risk information problem is not a deterrent to supply. The saving or capital accumulation aspect of pension contracts does not require information that is difficult to acquire. Adverse selection is a problem in that individuals with a propensity to live longer tend to be aware of the fact. But this is well recognised within the actuarial profession. Similarly, moral hazard does not pose a major problem, apart from a relatively small number of fraudulent claims. Risk concentration is also low; it is unlikely that a series of major medical breakthroughs will occur which will dramatically prolong life for a large section of the population.

Therefore in the field of retirement provision, there are no significant constraints on the private sector being a major or indeed the sole supplier. We are not discussing here the separate question of whether individuals can afford to buy adequate pensions, only the question of supply.

Private health and long-term care

The information needed to price health insurance is more difficult than in the case of pension provision. However, since insurance companies have been providing private health insurance contracts for many years, they have been building up databases on which they can 'fairly' price different types of health care contracts.

Adverse selection is a potential problem in that those with health problems may not fully disclose the information to insurers when they seek to purchase health insurance in order for appropriate prices to be charged. Insurance companies can have screening systems (e.g. medical tests) in order to reduce this problem in practice.

Moral hazard in the field of health care financing is a key issue. Moral hazard here arises from two sources:

- The problem of overuse by consumers.
- The problem that the providers of health care services overcharge or are profligate in the provision of services.

One has only to look at the cost of private health care in the US to realise the moral hazard problems involved. Insurance companies have the experience in designing contracts which can contain moral hazard. Controlling the moral hazard in the supply of health care services is more difficult, since it requires agreeing tariffs of charges and setting up monitoring systems. Of course, the large health insurance providers have the resources, especially collectively, to own private hospitals.

The provision of extensive private health insurance does not pose any undue problems for the insurance sector. One has only to look at Germany and Switzerland, where private health insurance, if mainly on a group basis, is a major area of business. Although health insurance is not purely private in Germany, there is considerably greater pluralism in its provision.

Private long-term care insurance is not a problem in principle and is provided in a number of EU countries. On the whole there is sufficient information to price the risk, and the analysis of available information is improving. Where information is limited, insurers have alternative methods of pricing. For example, part of the risk can be passed back to the customer by selling a product which pays a benefit limited in cash terms. This does not necessarily matter, as much of the risk can still be insured, particularly if the insurance is taken out some time before care is required. Adverse selection and moral hazard are not generally problems if proper medical evidence is requested and proper claims control is used. Individuals will not generally find the benefit of use if they are not actually in need of care. Cash-limiting the benefit can also be used as a mechanism to reduce adverse selection and moral hazard. Risk concentration is not generally a problem. However, insurance companies might be vulnerable to sudden changes in medical technology (for example, changes which significantly increased the life expectancy of people who were sick or disabled).

Conclusion on product potential

In summary, private insurance markets could in principle be suppliers in nearly all major areas in which social security provision currently exists. The only area that would appear to pose problems of supply is unemployment insurance. Lack of adequate information to have a 'fair' pricing system is a general obstacle, and, while short-term insurance (e.g. up to one year) supply is feasible if this information problem can be resolved, there are serious doubts about whether long-term unemployment insurance could be supplied, because of the problem of moral hazard. These problems may be eased through product design.

Issues in new product development

Let us now look at some product development issues associated with greater private sector provision. In the first place, because the underlying purpose behind social security is income maintenance (broadly defined), this provides a concept around which insurance companies could design new products and indeed package them together. The packaging of income-maintenance insurances would appear to be a promising direction. It is a common commercial practice for insurance companies to package various insurances within one contract. For example, household insurance consists of a package of property and liability insurances. From the standpoint of an insurance company, the packaging of insurances has two main benefits. First, it reduces the marketing costs. Second, it is possible for insurance companies to widen the coverage provided to customers. For example, an individual who is a serious health risk might find difficulty in purchasing a separate insurance policy for health insurance, or one that he considered to be affordable, but he would find it easier if it were part of a wider package, which included pensions, disability insurance, etc. This is because the insurance company is being offered a more diversified portfolio of risks.

Another difference between insurance contracts, as we have discussed, is that some insurance contracts entail funding and some do not. Another way of looking at this is that some contracts are long-term in nature and some are short-term. Contracts that involve funding are by their nature long-term contracts, whereas those concerned mainly with insurance protection rather than saving are conventionally short-term, usually one year. Hence the packaging of income-maintenance contracts also raises the issue of how one would combine long-term contracts, such as pensions, with short-term contracts, such as health insurance. The logical approach is to extend insurance contracts which are currently supplied on a short-term basis into long-term contracts. Such a development would be in line with the current marketing thinking within a number of insurance companies. These insurance companies are looking at new products which will allow a longer-term relationship with consumers to develop. Longer-term contracts have the benefit of reduced marketing and administration costs and also offer the customer wider, more flexible and more integrated insurance protection. They can also lead to proper funding of insurances such as health and long-term care.

Moreover, combining funded products and non-funded products (insurance-intensive products) also has financing benefits. Within a package, funded products generate the capital which can provide the intertemporal financing of insurance-intensive products. What happens in conventional short-term insurance is that the pooling of premiums across policyholders (i.e. savings) allows the risks of the individual to be financed by others through a process of cross-sectional support. The accumulation of saving within a long-term funded product can be used instead, at least in part, to finance these insurance-intensive products; the fact that these insurance-intensive products would now be packaged within long-term contracts means that the funded part of the package can be guaranteed to recover its financing costs over time.

The above would suggest that the insurance market product response to any greater potential role for them in gradually replacing current social security systems would most likely be in the form of a packaging of income-protection insurances within longer-term contracts. A distinction needs to be drawn between insurance supplied through personal policies and that supplied through group policies. There is greater potential for longer-term contracts through personal policies. Such a product solution would be similar to that which currently exists within the social security system itself: a packaging of contingent payment through an implicit long-term contract between the state and the individual. Group products may, however, also present a viable way forward (see below). There is unlikely to be one universal market solution: solutions will vary with the particular context in a given country and with consumer preferences. There are likely to be assurance and savings contracts supplied on both an individual and a group basis. Similarly, some products will be bought in a package while others will be purchased separately. But the common feature will be that the contracts are long-term.

PERCEIVED PROBLEMS OF MARKET PROVISION

. . . One of the problems which might be perceived by more market provision of insurance (particularly what might be termed 'social insurances' such as unemployment insurance) is the difficulty of uninsurability. The difficulty may become more acute with the advent of genetic testing. In making the move towards the privatisation of insurable risks, it is important to find a satisfactory method of dealing with the problem. One of the ways the market has of dealing with the problem is through the development of long-term contracts. Thus, for example, under the normal system of paying for health insurance in the UK, through renewable annual premiums, as somebody contracts a particular illness, or as somebody becomes old, their premiums may increase. However if, as in life insurance, a level premium were paid for an increasing risk, in a long-term contract the problem of uninsurability may not arise most of the time. There may still be some who are uninsurable (perhaps because of a condition that they have had since birth). There are ways that the state can deal with these problems without developing a comprehensive and all-encompassing social insurance system. For example, the state could subsidise private insurance premiums for some groups. Alternatively, as occurs in some states in the US motor insurance market, the state could divide the 'uninsurable' risks between insurance providers, forcing them to take on uneconomic risks which will be cross-subsidised by the better risks. This would be an effective way, for example, of dealing with those who were disabled from birth. It should also be noted that private insurances arranged under group schemes permit some degree of cross-subsidisation and more acceptance of 'uninsurable' risks than insurances arranged on an individual basis.

Moral hazard is also a problem which arises with private insurance. However, the authors would contend that this is a greater problem in state social insurance schemes. Private insurers will develop ways of dealing with moral hazard (for example, waiting periods before benefits are paid, no-claim discounts, deductibles, etc.) and can develop their own methods of claims control (for example, for unemployment insurance). These, in fact, are likely to be more successful than methods used by the state to control unreasonable claims and to prevent behaviour which is likely to increase claim frequency. Additionally, the private sector often has premium discounts for people who take precautions, which are likely to reduce claim frequency.

Private insurance is sometimes perceived as expensive and out of the reach of some individuals. This is best taken as two separate points. Administrative expenses of particular insurances can sometimes seem expensive relative to the administrative costs of running the social insurance system. This is unsurprising, as the social insurance system is providing a uniform benefit which is not tailored to individual consumers' needs. Nevertheless, the issue of the administrative costs of private insurance is important. The problem could, in fact, be alleviated if the government reduced its intervention in a number of areas:

- Reduced regulation (particularly of the selling process) would reduce costs significantly.
- A simplification of tax breaks would reduce the costs of product design and allow more competition between different methods of protecting against contingencies.
- The development of private provision in a number of fields may lead to the development of policies which cover a number of risks. This is likely to be cheaper.

In addition, if there was increased awareness of the need to insure (and possibly a degree of compulsion in some fields) this would reduce marketing costs. A significant proportion of expenses in private insurance markets arises from claims control and payment. The costs of this can be hidden in state insurance systems. Often, claims control will be less sophisticated in state systems but there will be more fraudulent claims. This is a hidden cost of state-provided insurance.

The point about private insurance being out of the reach of some individuals is more difficult to deal with. There is currently cross-subsidy between those on higher incomes and those on lower incomes because national insurance and taxes are broadly proportionate to income but the benefits that the system provides decrease, as a proportion of income, as income increases. However, the problem may not be as great as it may seem. One of the main causes of low income is that people are harmed by the very insurable events about which we are talking: insurance can protect against low income. Nevertheless, a movement to private insurance may put protection out of the reach of those on low incomes. There is much that can be done to alleviate this problem. For example, voucher systems ensure that all have insurance funded by, but not necessarily provided by, the state. Indeed, many areas of partnership could be developed which shared out the finance and provision of social insurance differently from the present situation. Tax systems can also be adjusted to help those who are affected by the movement towards more market insurance provision or direct payments can be made to insurance providers for those on low incomes (for example, to build up a pension fund).

It is also sometimes perceived that private insurance markets will deal badly with catastrophes and accumulations of risk. On the contrary there is every evidence that private markets can deal with these problems better than state insurance can. Private insurers have systems of reserving, diversification and reinsurance which can be used to reduce the risk of an accumulation of risks and claims. Very often, as is happening in continental Europe at the present time and as happened in the UK in the last recession, state insurance leads to an uncontrollable increase in claims and state spending. In private systems, premiums may rise after a cyclical increase in claims (for example, with mortgage indemnity insurance after the late 1980s) but if the increase in claims proves to be temporary, competition can pull premiums back down again.

Group products

Some of the problems of private insurance can be overcome by the development of group products. Indeed, group products have long been a way in which insurers have provided for those on low incomes. Group products require everyone in the group to take out a uniform product. They do reduce anti-selection risks considerably, because a condition of the contract can include that the vast majority of the group must insure. An average premium appropriate to the group can then be charged. Group insurances can also develop methods of claims screening, as the group can be big enough for the controller of the group to develop screening mechanisms (for example, in group health insurance, the overprovision of services can be monitored more easily than with individual health insurance). Group insurances can also significantly reduce transactions and marketing costs. Groups are normally centred on the workplace, although there is no reason why, in principle, other groups with common interests should not take out insurances.

Diverse institutions

The provision of social insurance has stifled the development of new products; we should therefore look not just at the existing product range when determining whether these insurances can be provided privately: such a focus would be too narrow. Similarly, we should not just look at existing market leaders in insurance when considering the relationship between insurer and insured which might exist if there were more private insurance. Markets, if they are allowed to, can innovate to find new solutions to insurance problems. Some of the solutions may involve the further development of institutions which have been stifled in the latter part of this century. Others may involve the development of completely new types of institution.

Friendly societies provided a range of services, to those of all income groups, in a way which combined genuine compassion with viable private insurance products. Indeed, Ernest Marples, speaking at the centenary congress of the Institute of Actuaries in 1948, expressed concern about the impact of social insurance schemes on modern civilisation. He predicted that social insurance would break down the mechanisms by which those who are not so well off could obtain insurance in a funded and secure way. Mr Marples also suggested that friendly societies had provided a Christian way by which security could be provided and that 'The national schemes were overriding all those earlier systems of private and individual enterprise.' It may be the case that some of those institutions will revive. However, the point is that the market is capable of discovering a whole range of institutions which meet consumer need. Those institutions can cover a whole spectrum of corporate structures: the only alternative to state-owned, controlled and financed institutions is not a wholly commercial organisation. Some examples of the products and institutions available in today's market are given below.

Insurance products can protect people from unemployment, or the consequences of accident, sickness and unemployment. Policies covering unemployment are available at between £3 and £3.75 monthly premium per £100 of monthly mortgage bill protected. The accident, sickness and unemployment cover is available at between £3.14 and £6.75 monthly premium. Typically these policies have a thirty-day waiting period before benefits become payable, and benefit lasts for twelve months.

Critical illness cover provides a large cash sum to help people carry on with their lives if diagnosed with a serious illness. There are 160 policies on offer in the UK. A recent innovative combined policy from Zurich Municipal includes life insurance, critical illness cover, permanent health insurance and unemployment protection in one policy. The term policy and critical illness cover provide a lump sum to pay off a mortgage in case of death or diagnosis of a life-threatening disease, whilst illnesses that prevent a policyholder from working are covered in addition to unemployment protection.

Insurance principles help millions of motorists and home owners to guard against risk. Eighteen million motorists are members of motoring organisations. The largest, the AA, now has 9.2 million members and about 2 million customers: the 11 million total is around double the number of people who are now members of trade unions. The RAC covers another 6 million members.

Competitive entry means that a plethora of services including Green Flag, Britannia and Europe Assist now compete to offer products ranging from roadside assistance at £35 per annum to £122 for a package including car hire, accommodation costs or transport home. Some policies offer no-claim bonuses – like the RAC's £25 'no call-out' discount at renewal – and others limit the number of call-outs.

Motoring organisations and water companies now offer home assistance policies where householders are guaranteed a fast response by tradesmen to household emergencies. For a premium of around £95 Thames Water Home Assist, for example, gives twenty-four-hour call-out within ninety minutes with up to three hours of labour and £100 of materials covering blocked or leaking pipes, faulty immersion heaters, windows, doors, locks, boilers and a miscellany of household problems. There is no limit to the number of call-outs per year.

Millions of people are already comfortable with the habit of using insurance solutions in their daily lives. There is now an opportunity for the insurance industry to reach out to them with a new range of products that could privatise large tracts of health and welfare provision, introduce competition, guarantee standards and ensure that funds are there to meet need as it arises. In the authors' view, there is no doubt that many insurances could be provided more effectively by semi-commercial organisations such as mutuals than by either purely commercial organisations or by the state. The former provide choice, opportunity and innovation more effectively than state-provided insurance can. On the other hand, they can give members the benefit of knowing that they 'belong' to and own the mutual organisation: something which, in the social insurance field, may be important. Many of the perceived problems of private provision can be overcome by the development of diverse institutions. Examples of such initiatives exist in the market.

PRIVATE PROVISION OF PENSIONS, HEALTH AND LONG-TERM CARE

In most EU countries, pension systems are in an acute state of crisis. The traditions of state-provided pensions are different across the EU. Appropriate approaches to reform may therefore vary. For example, a country where there is a tradition of the state providing pensions in a formal scheme with very little private provision may find it more difficult to reduce state pension promises. (On the other hand, the need for reform may be more acute.) A country, such as the UK, with significant private provision would find it less appropriate to introduce what will be termed a 'Chilean-style' reform which includes compulsory provision and the explicit buying out of state promises. In this section we will propose mechanisms of reform for different types of long-term insurance, describe the kinds of situation where particular reforms will be appropriate and give examples of countries which might benefit from different reforms. We will also discuss the ways in which the private sector could fill in any developing gaps in state provision. It is likely that most countries will find it appropriate to approach reform from a number of directions at the same time, in order to minimise the political impact.

With regard to pensions, in considering who should be the gainers and losers from any reform, it is necessary to consider how the social security debt has been built up. The debt could be regarded as being made up of two parts. The sum of those two parts is the total actuarial value of all commitments made to the current working and pensioner generations. That is the total unfunded liability. This total debt can be divided into the difference between the value of the benefits committed to current contributors and the value of the contributions of those taxpayers who will pay those benefits if the system remains on a pay-as-you-go basis, assuming that the contribution rates remain at the current level; and, second, the value of the contributions which are to be paid to meet the committed benefits, assuming that contributions remain at the current level.

It is useful to make this distinction because there are important political implications for the way in which we might deal with developing private provision. The first debt is, in a sense, the debt caused by the generation coming up to retirement not having enough children and living too long. As far as possible, the authors believe that social insurance systems should be altered so that, at worst, contribution levels do not increase. We believe that it is wholly wrong that the next generation should pay higher contributions in order to meet the benefits the coming beneficiary generation has promised to itself, without making proper provision. It would be unreasonable, however, to expect the generation of coming beneficiaries to bear the whole cost of the social insurance debt, regardless of the desirability of any move to a funded system. The first generation was the generation which benefited without having made any contribution. We should not necessarily wind up a pay-as-you-go scheme and expect that one particular generation should pay twice over.

This is a very important reason for having a number of strands to any reform. One of the problems of the Chilean model, discussed below, is that the current generation of contributors explicitly pays twice. It pays the taxes to meet the obligations made to the coming beneficiaries; it also funds its own pensions. The aim of reform should be to ensure that contributions to state schemes should not rise from current levels and that benefits are eroded gradually, so that, over a number of generations, funded provision is developed. Different ways of pursuing this aim are discussed below.

Reforming state pension schemes

Governments should, as far as possible, make a commitment not to increase the social insurance contribution rates in respect of pensions. The clear injustice of one generation having to meet commitments made by a previous generation would then end. It would be clear to those in the system that there were risks which had to be borne by the people in the social insurance system and that they might have to put extra resources aside in order to fund extra provision, in the event that state provision proved insufficient. If a constant contribution rate commitment was entered into, the demographic risks would be borne by the generation which determined the benefit levels, rather than by the succeeding generation, which currently pays for any commitments made by its predecessors. It is felt that any benefit cuts will be more palatable if they come with a commitment to cap contribution rates.

An interesting method of partially achieving a similar result as a constant contribution rate commitment was suggested by Hagemann and Nicoletti (1989). They suggested that, where social security taxes were largely paid by the employee, benefits should be defined in terms of pay net of social security taxes, rather than in terms of gross pay. This would mean that, if social security taxes increased owing to demographic pressures, benefit payments would immediately be reduced. This would have the effect of controlling costs but also of spreading the effects of a low birth rate across the population as a whole, including the retired population. Germany has taken this step to some extent.

If there is going to be a general aim to keep contribution rates from increasing and to decrease them over time, measures will need to be taken to reduce benefits. The measures can take three forms. First, we can reduce benefits explicitly (for example, by reducing the pension fraction); second, we can reduce benefits implicitly (for example, by raising the retirement age); third, we can reduce benefits in a way which spreads the cost over many generations (for example, by linking pensions to prices rather than earnings). All these approaches may be necessary in order to cap contribution rates and to facilitate the gradual movement to funded provision over many generations.

Such measures have already been taken in a number of countries in both Eastern and Western Europe. The state pension retirement age has been increased in Germany, Sweden and the UK (by equal-ising retirement ages for men and women at age sixty-five). This would normally need to be phased in if it was going to be politically acceptable and not create 'policy uncertainty' amongst those who are close to retirement age. Raising the retirement age gradually has the advantage of spreading the cost of adjustment over a number of generations. However, it is unlikely to promote funded provision, as people will still rely on the state and carry on working until the later retirement age. Hagemann and Nicoletti (1989) demonstrated the extent of the possible savings from an increase in retirement age in Germany and Sweden. A modest increase of two years could lower social security tax rates by between 3 per cent and 4 per cent.

The UK and a number of other EU countries have changed the formula by which the pension is calculated. The most common way to do this is by applying a given pension fraction to final average salary but the averaging is done over a greater number of years (for example, the best twenty years, rather than the best three years). This method can be used to reduce the pension significantly. Again, a method has to be found of phasing in any such reform. The best approach is probably to increase the number of years used to calculate the final pension gradually over a generation. It would be relatively easy to phase in such a reform so that the full benefit to finances was felt by 2030, when most state pension schemes reach their crisis point.

State pension benefits could be linked to prices instead of earn-ings. This has been done in the UK. This leads to the pension falling relative to earnings. The advantage of this type of reform is that it has its own mechanism of gradual phasing in (as cumulative increases in prices gradually slip behind cumulative increases in earnings). Thus, once the political decision is taken to break a link with earnings, the cost savings accumulate over time. If the link with earnings is never restored, this mechanism will ensure that the extent of the state pension scheme will reduce significantly over time (rather than just leading to a once-and-for-all reduction, as when the pension fraction is reduced).

A further reform of state schemes to limit benefits would be to put a cap on the level of earnings that could be considered when calculating the pension to be received. The earnings cap has two effects. It can produce an immediate reduction in the state benefit for those on high earnings. There will then be some incentive for such people to make personal funded provision. Second, if the cap is not linked to average earnings, it can be used to reduce gradually the extent of the state scheme as earnings increase over time and make the earnings cap relevant to more people.

Opting out of long-term insurances

We would also like to see wide-ranging opting out of state-provided insurance benefits encouraged. EU governments should develop innovative ways of allowing their citizens to insure a number of risks privately whilst opting out of state provision. This opting out should be on actuarially neutral grounds so that there is no net cost to the state of allowing the opt-out. Individuals should be able to opt out of any state-provided pension, life insurance or widows' benefit, with the state allowing a reduced contribution into the national scheme. Such opting out could be extended to a number of benefits. The state could give a tax allowance to people who take out private health or long-term care insurance at a reasonably early age, paying level annual premiums for life, as long as the private contracts provide the benefits which would otherwise have been provided by the state. With 'baseline' benefits such as health insurance, the minimum level of state pension, etc., the state will need to lay down stricter qualifying conditions, because the state would have to meet the cost if the policy failed to provide the benefit. Other insurable risks (unemployment insurance, disability insurance, etc.) could also be allowed for opting out.

Opting out has a very similar effect to vouchers, because the government determines the minimum amount of income which is spent on a particular service whilst giving freedom as to how it is spent. However, opting out can destabilise pay-as-you-go pension systems, in the same way that the so-called 'Chilean' solution to the pensions problem (described below) does. It effectively requires the whole debt to be met over two generations, although this is the case only with respect to that part of the population which does opt out. To illustrate the point, consider a twenty-one-year-old who has just started making contributions to the state scheme. His contributions are required to meet the pensions of the generations which are currently receiving pensions (as those pensions were not pre-funded). If this person 'opts out' and uses any rebate to set up a personal pension, the social insurance fund will appear to be in deficit. The 'opting out' generation will have to fund the deficit through higher taxes, thus paying twice for pension benefits. In practice, however, some of the implicit debt should in any case be met by the current generation of contributors, and this effect will be limited by the fact that only a proportion of the work force will opt out.

In some countries the above reforms may be sufficient to develop funded provision, particularly in pensions. The key is to ensure that unfunded provision is at a relatively restricted level and that all participants in the state schemes have an opportunity to develop alternative (as well as supplementary) private provision without having to pay twice for insurance services such as health care, long-term care and pensions. In a sense, the above proposals could be regarded as a traditional British Conservative approach to the problem. There would be no radical changes or restructuring but a series of controls and incentives created to gradually reduce the impending financial crisis and develop private provision. The multi-pillar and Chilean solutions are specifically intended to deal with pensions provision and are more appropriate in cases where the state scheme is all-encompassing, in serious financial trouble and/or where a tradition of paternalism exists within the country with regard to the provision of state benefits.

Creating a multi-pillar pension system

Many state pension schemes need rationalising so that it is clear what the state will and will not provide and so that a basis can be defined for determining the maximum benefits the state will offer to future contributors. Such a process is often described as creating a multi-pillared system. The first pillar could be a minimal level of state benefit and the second pillar could be compulsory but privately funded. The third pillar would be purely voluntary but with tax incentives to encourage further provision. The first pillar could be publicly financed on a pay-as-you-go basis and is mainly intended to ensure the level of income redistribution that is regarded as desirable: to ensure that old people enjoy a given basic standard of living. The first pillar could be means-tested, and this would cut costs. However, means-tested benefits lead to disincentives and can be complex to administer. In general terms, it is better to set up the public pillar with other cost control mechanisms so that means testing is not necessary. For example, the minimum level of pension should be indexed to prices and not to wages; the age at which the public pillar pension is paid should be constantly adjusted so that the life expectancy beyond that age remains approximately constant; and the level of pension paid under the public pillar should be limited and should perhaps be below social security subsistence levels (so that those who receive only the public pension may also be in receipt of means-tested benefits). It should be stressed that the public pillar is an absolute last resort for those who slip through all the other possible safety nets and, for some reason, do not have pensions from the other pillars. Alternatively, the first pillar could be a compulsory private, funded pillar with a state guarantee (as with the 1992–97 Conservative government's 'Basic Pension Plus' proposal).

If the second pillar is phased in (allowing those who have accrued benefits in the earnings-related state scheme to continue in the scheme), those who are making private provision should get a social insurance tax rebate, calculated on a fair actuarial basis.

For countries which already have two pillars (for example, Denmark, the UK, the Netherlands) the proposals above may just involve a tidying-up exercise. For countries such as Belgium, France and Italy, which have an extensive earnings-related first pillar, a substantial restructuring may be necessary. Such restructuring is vital if the goal of private pension provision is to be achieved and the financial crisis averted.

Kessler (1988) and Giarini (1990) have suggested that the social security burden could be eased by the development of four 'pillars'. The first three pillars relate to state and private formal pension provision. The fourth pillar relates to the ability of those who are retired to undertake part-time work to supplement their pension. This is a sensible approach, both because of the increasing labour shortage which will arise as the population ages and because those who are retired will be enjoying a longer and healthier retirement.

The 'Chilean' solution

It is likely that countries where the state scheme is very formal and where there is little private provision will have most difficulty reducing state benefits and encouraging private provision. In this case the so-called 'Chilean' solution may be appropriate. That solution has been proposed by some British Conservative commentators. However, the Chilean solution is not really necessary in the UK and would probably be more interventionist than the current system. The Chilean solution is, in fact, very paternalist. However, where the state has a monopoly of provision, it does facilitate a radical move to private provision, giving workers considerably more choice than they have currently. It recognises the implicit debt and makes the state face up to the problem of financing it. It also provides workers with an alternative mechanism of pension provision in which they can have confidence, as an alternative to state provision. The Chilean solution has two distinctive features.

In Chile the government turned implicit social security debt into explicit debt. The debt was made up of three components: first, the pensions of those who had retired; second, the pensions of those who had decided to remain with the state system, and, third, the pensions which had already been accrued by those who had decided to leave the state system when opting out was allowed. This third group was offered 'recognition bonds' equal to the present value of their accrued pension liabilities. The recognition bonds were non-transferable but, in other respects, were just like government bonds, and earned interest at 4 per cent above the rate of inflation. At retirement they were redeemed for lump-sum payments which could be made into the defined contribution pension fund accounts of the individuals. The recognition bonds therefore had two important features. They recognised as explicit the implicit social security debt and put an assessed value on that debt. Second, they were designed in a way which limited the cash-flow problems which could have been caused by simply issuing government bonds or making one-off immediate payments into individuals' pension schemes: this could have caused a loss of confidence in the bond market.

A good contrast with the Chilean solution has been provided by the UK approach and also by proposals by the Conservative Party's 'Basic Pension Plus' plan. The Conservative Party proposed the development of funding and private provision only for new entrants to the state scheme (as opposed to explicitly recognising existing liabilities). It also proposed a compulsory contribution up to a certain level, not up to a given proportion of salary. The compulsory contribution is therefore set at the minimum level necessary so that an individual will not be a burden to the state in old age. All provision above that level is voluntary. The earlier reforms of the State Earnings Related Pension Scheme had a similar approach, although opting out of the state scheme, in that case, was also voluntary. The voluntarism of the British approach sits neatly with the underlying philosophy of the British tradition. It also reflects the fact that the pensions problem has not reached 'emergency' proportions. Reform proposals from the 1997 Labour government are awaited. However, something closer to the Chilean approach may be more appropriate in other EU countries.

One advantage of the Chilean approach is that it makes implicit debt explicit. This explicit debt could be partially extinguished and the recognition bonds partially redeemed by the proceeds from the privatisation of state industries. Indeed, this makes economic sense. The state would then be privatising its assets and liabilities simultaneously. This approach would also alleviate cash-flow problems.

Private provision in respect of other risks which can be pre-funded: health care and long-term care for the elderly

When considering the development of private markets in health care, the issues are somewhat different from those related to pensions. The most important issue facing most developed countries, as far as pensions are concerned, is the funding issue. With regard to health care, the funding issues, if health care is taken alone, are not as significant. However, providing choice, variety, efficiency in provision and innovation are all very important. Some of the advantages of the development of private provision can therefore be provided with a voucher system: see Bassett (1993). A voucher system ensures that public funding remains but that people have more choice about the type of care that they consume. It also ensures that those who choose to insure privately do not pay for their health care twice. Tax relief on health care premiums can also achieve the same objectives for a limited number of people who choose to take out private insurance and take advantage of the tax relief.

Regarding long-term care, in some countries, such as Germany, there is compulsory long-term care insurance. In the UK long-term care provision is means-tested. . . . It is clear that long-term care is an insurable risk. However, most people in the UK do not finance the provision of long-term care by taking out insurance. Some finance it by house sale and some by saving (possibly followed by house sale if the savings run out). Many others receive care informally, provided by friends and relatives. The UK government faces two main problems. One is that many of those who 'fail' the means test and have to sell their house resent having to do so: there is a consequent addition to the poverty trap, because those who do not own assets have their long-term care financed by the state. The second problem is that, despite the fact that, in principle, individuals have to fund their own care, subject to the means test, there is a growing burden falling on the state.

The 1992–97 Conservative government proposed an increase in social security means-testing limits where people take out their own insurance. This was likely to lead to the government paying for more care than was previously the case. However, it might encourage more private insurance. An alternative would be to offer some kind of favourable tax treatment of long-term care policies. The arguments in favour of this are discussed in Booth (1996). A danger of compulsory fully insured systems (whether provided by the state or the private sector) is that they lead to the breakdown of all forms of care which are not free at the point of use (including informal care). This could be very expensive and lead to very high insurance premiums or social security taxes. Compulsory or state insurance for long-term care is making a particular type of insurance compulsory when, in fact, given a free choice, people like to provide for care in a variety of ways. The authors do not believe that it is appropriate to promote long-term care insurance through compulsion.

Policy conclusions on private provision

We would conclude that there are many areas where private insurance institutions could take over from the state in the provision of social insurance. However, we should not rely on the current institutions and products to fulfil the market need. Before private insurance can evolve, consumers need to know what cover they will get from the state social insurance system. In the fields of health, unemployment, long-term care and disability the state should announce what its long-term intentions are. In health, users of the NHS in the UK should know precisely what services it will provide and what reasonable waiting times and 'hotel-type' facilities will be available. The state should make a contract with the people so that policy uncertainty is ended and people can make their own decisions about taking out supplementary insurance in a climate of long-term certainty. In sensitive areas such as health and long-term care we believe that governments should have an open mind towards the involvement of private insurance institutions. There is no reason why the finance, the management of the insurance risk and the provision of the service should all come from the government. The needs of those on both high and low incomes might be better served if the boundaries between state and private provision were drawn differently.

In pensions, continental EU countries need to review their arrangements with great urgency to reduce the cost of state pensions and encourage funded provision. There may need to be an explicit 'buying out' of state pension arrangements and compulsion for private provision, as in the Chilean model. In the UK there is less urgency but the development of further funded provision, particularly for the low-paid, would be an advantage.

NOTES

This chapter is reprinted by permission of the European Policy Forum from its pamphlet *The Insurance Solution* (London, 1997).

1 Broadly speaking, the actuarial value of the unfunded benefits could be regarded as the amount which needs to be invested today to meet the benefits that are expected to be paid to future generations.

REFERENCES

The Actuary (1996) *The Actuary* (magazine of the actuarial profession), vols 6/7, Actuarial Society, Staple Inn, London.
Bassett M. (1993) *A Health Cheque for All: Proposals for a Mixed Market in Health Care*, European Policy Forum, London.
Besseling P. J. and Zeeuw R. F. (1993) *The Financing of Pensions in Europe: Challenges and Opportunities*, Centre for European Policy Studies Report 14, CEPS.
Booth P. M. (1996) *The Long-term View: Financing Care for the Elderly*, Politeia, London.

Booth P. M. and Stroinski K. (1996) 'The joint development of the insurance and investment markets in Poland', *British Actuarial Journal* 2, 3: 741–63.

Brown R. L. (1995) 'Paygo funding stability and intergenerational equity', *SCOR Notes.*

Chand S. K. and Jaeger A. (1996) *Ageing Populations and Public Pension Schemes,* International Monetary Fund Occasional Paper 147, IMF, Washington, D.C.

de la Fuente R. (1995) *An Ageing Europe: The Implications for Financial Markets,* Banque Paribas, London.

De Ryck K. (1996) *European Pension Funds: Their Impact on European Capital Markets and Competitiveness,* European Federation for Retirement Provision.

Financial Times (1996) *Insurance in the EU, Switzerland and Norway 1996: Structures of the Financial Markets,* London: FT Financial Publishing.

Franco D. and Munzi T. (1996) *Public Pension Expenditure Prospects in the European Union: A Survey of National Projections,* European Economy Reports and Studies 3, European Commission, Brussels.

Giarini O. (1990) 'Introduction: the opportunities of the four pillars strategy', *Geneva Papers on Risk and Insurance* 50.

Hagemann R. P. and Nicoletti G. (1989) *Population Ageing: Economic Effects and some Policy Implications for Financing Public Pensions,* OECD Economic Studies 12, OECD, Paris.

Hayek F. A. (1945) *The Road to Serfdom,* London: Routledge and Kegan Paul.

Kessler D. (1988) 'The four pillars of retirement', *Geneva Papers on Risk and Insurance* 49.

Kessler D. (1996) 'Preventing Conflicts between the Generations', twentieth annual lecture of the Geneva Association, London.

Lindbeck A. (1994) 'Uncertainty under the welfare state: policy-induced risk', *Geneva Papers on Risk and Insurance* 73.

Paribas (1995) *Economic Brief* 18 December, Paribas Capital Markets, London.

Roseveare D., Leibfritz W., Fore D. and Wurzel E. (1996) *Ageing Populations, Pension Systems and Government Budgets: Simulations for Twenty OECD Countries,* OECD Economics Department Working Paper 168, OECD, Paris.

Seldon A. (1981) *Whither the Welfare State?* Institute of Economic Affairs Occasional Paper 60, IEA, London.

Seldon A. *et al.* (1996) *Re-privatising Welfare: After the Lost Century,* Institute of Economic Affairs Readings 45, IEA, London.

Skrabski A. (1996) 'What kind of pension system does the average Hungarian want?', *Hungarian Federation of Mutual Funds Newsletter,* April, pp. 3–4.

Taverne D. (1995) *The Pension Time Bomb in Europe,* Federal Trust Report, The Federal Trust.

Walker B. W. (1991) *The Funding of Health Care in the Year 2000,* Proceedings of the 1991 Institute of Actuaries of Australia Hobart Convention, Institute of Actuaries of Australia.

11

ASSURANCE, PENSIONING AND LONG-TERM CARE

Peter G. Moore

The UK financial services sector has been in a state of flux ever since the so-called 'Big Bang': the moment in the 1980s when the financial services markets were liberalised. Traditional segmentation of these markets has been steadily eroded, and many businesses are confronted with new competitors who are not at all like themselves, and who operate within radically different cost structures and follow unexpected or unfamiliar strategies. The markets, and the key players involved, are becoming more global, whilst the assurance industry is concentrating into a smaller set of 'mega' companies, each operating in the various major markets. Capacity has become highly mobile and is readily redistributed into markets that offer either high profitability or faster growth, or both. Such changes have caused increasing uncertainty and instability. The life cycles of products, companies and even entire industries are growing shorter. Traditionally profitable products are becoming less so, squeezing the industry's long-term return on capital and undermining the incentives to devise in-service improvements, new products or lowered business expenses. In pursuit of greater profits, corporations, and effectively their customers, sometimes take unprecedented risks with extremely complex, unproven products (e.g. the so-called 'derivatives' that brought down the house of Baring).

Against this backdrop, life assurance companies have scrambled to adapt. There has been a rush into 'tied' distribution relationships with banks, building societies and other financial institutions. The mix of business would, and has, been changed, with pension, single premium and unit trust products growing substantially in importance. There have been many mergers and diversifications (e.g. into estate agencies), and foreign imitations. For the most part, the responses have been reactive rather than anticipatory, tactical rather than strategic, perceived rather than systematic, and evolutionary rather than revolutionary.

What follows in this chapter is a consideration of the evolution in the UK of the insurance industry's involvement in pensions. Morally speaking, this involvement has left much to be desired. The relatively recent marketing of new pension products has left many customers worse off than they would have been, and efforts to compensate customers for bad advice have not always covered losses. Longerstanding ethical problems in private pension provision have also not been entirely overcome. The entitlement to pension benefits of divorced women is a case in point. There has, again, long been an undue burden on prospective pensioners if they change their job often. Gradual changes in the form of private sector pensions may not protect individuals from the effects of inflation.

Despite these problems, there is no evident alternative to an increasing role for insurance companies, and those managing pension schemes generally, in the provision of pensions. Public sector pension schemes around the world are hugely overextended financially, and will become intolerably overextended in the future. For similar reasons, the public provision of long-term care for the elderly may come to be unaffordable without the involvement of the insurance industry. The moral case for private involvement may as well be considerable. Under current arrangements, means testing confiscates the savings of the prudent while rewarding those who have counted on the state to come to the rescue in their old age.

PENSIONING RESPONSIBILITIES: THE STATE'S, THE EMPLOYER'S OR THE INDIVIDUAL'S?

The suggestion that the responsibility for pensions lies with business or the state as opposed to individuals, is in a sense fanciful. Whether retirement income is funded by current taxation through levies from employment earnings, or through savings (forced or voluntary), individuals in the end have to pay. It is important, though, to devise a mechanism or mechanisms that are most likely to ensure that the largest possible number of people enjoy an adequate income in retirement. Such a mechanism must generate a system of pensioning that is adequate, fair and equitable to all concerned. At the same time the cost must not become an intolerable burden

Table 11.1 Life expectation of males aged sixty

Country	1960	1970	1980	1990	1994
UK	11.9	12.0	12.6	14.1	14.7
France	12.5	13.0	14.0	15.6	16.2

Source: Eurostat, 1996.

on taxpayers, their children or even their grandchildren. A successful pension scenario depends upon demography, which is largely determined in advance, allied to the appropriate availability of adequate financial resources.

The age structure of a future population is largely dependent on two factors: the rate of mortality and the rate of fertility. On the former, rates of mortality are to a large degree predictable, and life expectancy in years for males reaching sixty-five (the common pension age) is shown in Table 11.1.

The figures for females are approximately two-and-a-half years higher than for males. Moreover, for both sexes the expectation of life is rising steadily, which makes higher demands on the pension costs for those retiring at sixty-five (or at an earlier age).

An Elderly Dependence Ratio is also relevant. This ratio is defined as the number of persons aged sixty-five-plus, expressed as a percentage of the number of persons in the age group fifteen to sixty-four. These ratios, and their current projections, are shown in Table 11.2. In broad terms the Elderly Dependence Ratio is expected almost to double in the next fifty years. This inevitably has serious implications in terms of pensioning provision, e.g. whether a higher basic pension age may be required in order to rebalance the ratio of pensioners to workers.

The state's direct role in UK pensions has remained relatively limited in recent years. This is in contrast to the greater role that is played by state pensions in other large European countries such as France, Germany and Italy. In those three countries the state is

Table 11.2 Elderly Dependence Ratio, current and projected

Country	1995	2000	2010	2020	2030	2050
UK	24.3	24.4	25.8	31.2	38.7	41.2
France	22.1	23.6	24.6	32.3	39.1	43.5

Source: Bos *et al.* (1994).

the main provider of retirement income, either directly, or indirectly through the sponsorship of industry-managed systems (the French *répartition* system, for example).

The UK flat-rate Retirement Pension Scheme and the allied UK State Earnings Retirement Pension Scheme (SERPS) operate on a pay-as-you-go principle. No funds are built up and managed; rather the state pays annually for the pensions required from current taxation monies. The National Insurance or SERPS contribution is added to the Treasury's annual income.

This approach was introduced in many countries in the nineteenth century and it fitted the demographic pattern of the time. There were plenty of young men at work (full employment is a desirable condition for an appropriate pay-as-you-go system) and there were relatively few individuals aged sixty-five or more who were drawing a pension in relation to those still working. Demography has, however, turned full circle as countries have become more developed, particularly for those which established national pay-as-you-go schemes and now find that, with lower birth rates and greater longevity, pension provision has become extremely expensive to the state.

Many developed countries have now huge outstanding unfunded public budget liabilities. Present calculations from the OECD suggest that, by 2003, France will have unfunded public budget liabilities of 103 per cent of its GDP; Germany 105 per cent; and Italy 146 per cent. Japan is even worse, at 314 per cent. The UK, by contrast, is enjoying a modest 'profit' (always provided, of course, that it makes no adverse changes in its present pension policies which involve substantial private funded pension provisions).

The World Bank makes it clear that the state in virtually all developed countries is having to retreat from its role as a major provider of retirement income. Individuals will have to take more responsibility for themselves. When governments seek to offload social costs such as pensions they – perhaps naturally – turn first to employers to fill the gap. This then throws up the necessity for government to regulate the employers' handling of their employees' pensions with a mass of consequential legislation to protect individuals who may have had many employers over a career of forty years or more.

An overhaul of pensioning has been overdue in the UK for some years. Those who have had little pensioning beyond the state pension have found that, relative to earnings, the pension has steadily fallen. At one time the state pension had been 40 per cent of average earnings for a married couple. This has now fallen well below 30 per cent, and some 50 per cent of pensioners effectively have only the state pension on which to subsist. (Many such pensions can call upon some means-tested supplementary benefits). Since the state pension goes to all, the government tends to allow the state pension to drift, since the supplementary benefits are means-tested. The total cost of the state pension plus supplementary benefits rises more slowly than would a state pension indexed to changes in the percentage of average earnings (and not to the retail price index).

In the UK, pensioners in the private sector were shocked by the Maxwell scandal: funds ostensibly held in trust by the pension scheme to pay pensions were missing when Maxwell died. The subsequent litigation aimed at reducing such risks of fraud and insolvency, and to conform with modern standards of job mobility and self-determination. It did not, however, provide public money to assist lost cash from the Maxwell debacle itself.

Most people believe that pension balances (however defined and managed) ought to be as portable as possible, allowing employees to be able to contribute on a tax-deferred basis up to reasonably high limits on top of employers' contributions. This would encourage individual responsibility, leading to a higher national savings rate, which, in turn, would make it easier to provide better pensions. Self-management of pensions ought to be allowed, by providing, for example, a menu of unit trusts from which an individual's pension balances can be drawn. Financial institutions should be bonded and competitive as regards the costs of holding and managing unit trusts (or equivalent investments) and the costs of switching.

Consumer protection and product liability laws applicable to financial services should be strengthened. Standards of disclosure ought to be raised, linked with concepts of what consumers require in order to make 'informed decisions'. Misadvising should be more clearly transparent, as should be the dividing line between 'selling' and 'advising'. The nature of a company's responsibilities and liabilities as they affect the relationship with the consumer ought to be more transparent.

The government (any government) wants to off-load the cost of pensioning to individuals as far as it can, and does not want to find itself picking up the tab for those who have been improvident. At the same time UK legislation of pensions has become much less benign. Employers, or the insurance companies involved, are being forced to incur more costs in order to comply with the myriad new regulations – indeed, the regulations can now also involve litigation in courts outside the UK (e.g. the European Court of Justice).

Consequently some employers are moving away from defined benefit pension schemes towards defined contributions-based pensions where the benefits are not fixed in advance and both regulations and costs to the company are less onerous. The former types of pensioning provided considerable advantages to an employee, but do have some disadvantages, e.g. lack of mobility of pensions between different firms which have differing schemes. Employers in the UK who have been keen to retain the final salary approach may be in retreat, but a rearguard action has been strongly launched, particularly by the better paid employees in areas where jobs switches are relatively rare.

If a more individualistic approach with a new savings culture is to emerge under the Blair government, it will have to take action to remove barriers that give poor incentives to save. This means greater flexibility in Inland Revenue rules, a more realistic attitude to the myriad regulations, appropriate tax rebates and, above all, a severe pruning of the costs that arise in many forms of savings.

The general tremors within Europe as it switches over from pay-as-you-go schemes to funded schemes is moving in favour of money purchase systems rather than the defined benefit schemes popular in the UK. The French socialist government has not yet clarified its views but, as the law now stands, it clearly favours money purchase both in the social security provision and in the provision of pensions outside the government social security schemes. Tax approved limits in such countries are expressed in terms of contributions, not benefits.

The current law in Italy states that, for all new schemes, the money purchase approach is required. The case is the same in Spain. The apparent decline in the average length of tenure with any one employer, and the rise of part-time and alternative forms of employment, are trends generally viewed in Europe as favouring money purchase schemes.

Germany has had some difficulties in determining its pension provisioning, with its reinsurance contracts backing company reserves. But, with cession of the contracts to the individuals in the case of company insolvency, money purchase schemes are seen as an increasingly important route for general pension provision. Countries in Eastern Europe, such as the Czech Republic and Hungary, have both recently implemented such legislation.

The defined benefits 'club' is shrinking within Europe, so that the only members left are Ireland, the UK (partially), Belgium and

Germany (temporarily). The broad view is that there is an accelerating trend towards money purchase. One possible brake that may slow down the shift from defined benefit schemes concerns inflation. Over the course of a working life (commonly around forty years) defined benefit schemes could be harmed less by inflation than the alternative.

PENSIONS IN THE UK

The UK pension scene for the past twenty-five years has consisted primarily of a modest state pension for all. To this has been added either a company pension of a defined benefit type (DB), or a company pension of a defined contribution type (DC); or a further state pension via the State Earnings Retirement Pension Scheme (SERPS). All individuals who have worked should have accumulated some assets from at least one of these three possible additions and could, in some instances, have accumulated contributions from two or even all three such sources.

The state retirement pension, available to all who have worked and paid National Insurance contributions, is modest. Currently a married couple with a full record receive around £5,250 per annum, a single person £3,250 per annum. The pension is up-rated annually by the change in the retail prices index. Before 1980 the up-rating was based on the index of earnings, which, if it had been maintained, would now be giving such pensioners £6,750 per annum, or £5,200 per annum, respectively. These figures should be compared with the current level of average earnings of about £19,750 per annum. Nearly half of all current pensioners live solely on the state retirement pension plus, in many cases, some governmental means-tested income support top-up.

Defined benefit schemes currently involve about 45 per cent of employees, although this percentage is gradually falling. In a defined benefit (also referred to as a final salary) scheme the pension of the individual retiree is calculated, for example, by multiplying the salary immediately before retirement by a fraction (commonly eighteenths) linked to the number of years that the employee has worked for the company. Additionally a tax-free lump sum of three times the annual pension is commonly paid. The Inland Revenue regards the allowable maximum, including any lump sum, as two-thirds of final retirement salary with forty years of service to count. Thus, if the deal is, say, one-sixtieth of preretirement pay for each year of service, an employee who has thirty years under his or her belt could retire on half salary. Alternatively he or she in many schemes could retire with an annual pension of 37.5 per cent of final salary, plus a tax-free lump sum equal to 112.5 per cent of a year's final salary. Not many retirees, however, achieve a pension based on forty years of service from one employer. The tax-free lump sum on retirement is well entrenched, and much appreciated, but a hungry Chancellor of the Exchequer might one day be tempted to tax such a juicy morsel!

Crucially, the pension is fixed, except that annual upgrades on the basis of the change in the retail price index have, by law, to be added – up to a maximum of 5 per cent in any one year. Employers can voluntarily give employees a review up to the whole of the annual RPI change. A firm that has a DB scheme can offer membership to all its employees, but individuals cannot now always be forced to join. If an employee declines membership he or she must join either a personal pension scheme (i.e. a DC form of scheme) or become a member of SERPS. If an employee declines membership of the firm's scheme, the employer cannot be compelled to pass his normal DB scheme contribution to a DC scheme.

Defined benefit schemes have to be kept solvent. An independent actuarial evaluation of all such schemes has to be held at least once every three years. Should the fund fall below its solvency level the employer has to add more cash to the fund to make good any shortfall.

Final salary (DB) schemes have been a boon to many employees, but there can be drawbacks. Many employees switch companies and pension schemes, voluntarily or involuntarily, during their forty-year employment career. For those who switch there can be difficulties and pitfalls. Such employees can maintain a deferred pension with an earlier employer which is augmented by the RPI, but it will ignore the effects of rising salaries over time and age. Alternatively the employee can request to be given 'added years' when moving across to a new similar DB scheme. In practice the added years will be somewhat smaller in relation to total previous service. Commonly about 60 per cent of years worked are transferred, e.g. some ten years in the previous scheme may count as six years in the new scheme. A broad calculation suggests that, if an employee had four different employers, each with ten years' service, in his forty-year career, the final pension would be only about half the pension had the employee had all his service with a single firm (or rather a single pension scheme). The actuarial profession has recently suggested that DB transfer from one firm to another should be carried out on a new basis, referred to by actuaries as the Minimum Funding Requirement. Most actuaries now use this method, which involves an improvement on the pension calculations applicable to many transfers.

From an employer's point of view, the DB scheme relies heavily on fund managers being able to read the stock market well. Most employers have done a good job and many schemes have indeed accumulated surpluses from time to time. This, however, may not always be the case; a stock market collapse, or a fall with a slow recovery, can leave employers open to substantial liabilities. Valuations in the UK are primarily based upon the anticipated stream of dividend income, which is generally less volatile than a valuation of investment capital prices at a given date, as is customarily used in the US. The cost of administering a pension scheme is generally borne by the employer.

In 1988–89 there were some 10.8 million members in DB schemes, of which 6.0 million were in the private sector and 4.7 million in the public sector. However, by 1994–95 the total had fallen to 9.3 million, with 4.8 million in the private sector and 4.5 million in the public sector. The fall in the private sector has dropped further since 1994–95, and it is clear that there has been a swing, particularly in the private sector, from DB to deferred contribution (DC) or money purchase schemes. The government has recently placed a ceiling, currently £84,000, on the maximum amount that can be considered for earnings that are to be counted towards a DB pension scheme for any individual. The ceiling will be reached slowly but, as the limit is up-rated by the change in the index of retail prices rather than the index of earnings, it will in the long run involve many scheme members having their pension rights curtailed.

The Pension Act of 1995 allowed individuals to switch from a company scheme into a personal pension scheme. This encouraged mis-selling and, for most individuals concerned, such a switch has been a retrograde step. The individuals were commonly drawn from the public sector, where DB schemes were frequent. Some 1.5 million people were involved in all, of which around 900,000 are priority cases of mis-selling by pension companies offering personal pensions lower in amount than would have been the case with the DB route. Only about 5 per cent of the cases had, up to 1997, been resolved. Many of the individuals involved were wrongly advised by agents of pension companies to enter into a personal pension plan (i.e. into a DC plan). Companies with DB schemes ironically frequently gained financially through employees switching into a DC scheme as the employer's contribution became defunct.

The then government must accept part of the blame, since it instigated a mass media advertising campaign which, in many instances, convinced employees that a personal pension (DC) was superior to a defined benefit (DB) pension! Some insurance companies and financial advisers have made genuine efforts to compensate those involved but many companies, including some well known ones, are well behind schedule in rectifying the consequences of the poor advice given to employees.

Whilst the DB schemes of the private sector companies have been tightly regulated, the management of DB public sector schemes has been somewhat lax. Such public sector schemes include employees of the NHS, local government authorities, teachers, civil servants, fire services, police employees, etc. Some of these schemes involved are unfunded, i.e. there is no build-up of cash and pensions are paid as required from current income, the benefits having been delineated in advance; others, e.g. for teachers, are funded. Many individuals have been allowed special early retirement rights. This should automatically require extra revenue to be injected into the appropriate scheme to fund the extra cost but it has not always been done, thus financially weakening the scheme as a whole and raising costs to the government or local authority.

Two examples can be quoted. In recent years schoolteachers over the age of fifty could retire early with a pension based as if they had worked up to age sixty. No cash was required from the relevant local authority up front to pay for the pension fund to cover this special retirement and the extra cash requirement effectively fell on the government, i.e. the public. In the second case, the fire services anticipate that early retirements will, in ten years' time, require some 25 per cent of the total fire brigade annual budget to pay for their current pensions! The consequences of such anomalies in public sector DB schemes, which in the past have generally been run extremely well, have now reached crisis point. The pressure from management to cut staff and to give generous early retirements has not been allowed for in the funding.

The defined contribution (DC) or money purchase schemes, commonly referred to nowadays as personal pensions, are becoming more common. These schemes are seen as providing an alternative and more flexible type of pension arrangement. With these schemes it is the contributions that are fixed; the benefits can, and do, vary. Contributions are paid into a fund on a regular basis, earmarked for each individual and invested to build up a lump sum. This individual fund is used at retirement to buy an annuity to provide the requisite pension.

Individuals will normally choose the insurance company they wish to handle their pension accounts. This form of investment absolves the employer from a great deal of concern, with the added advantage that it is considered better suited to many modern employees' needs. Individuals with a DC scheme effectively have their own pot of invested cash so that shifting from one employer to another is a relatively straightforward matter. There are, however, drawbacks to such schemes. First, there is the cost of holding the cash with a legally authorised organisation which invests the funds and deals with the paperwork. In the early years, while the individual's fund builds up, the costs are relatively high and are siphoned off to the organiser – commonly an insurance company. Second, money purchase schemes are always at risk from stock market fluctuations. Most DB schemes commonly invest a total of 15–20 per cent of annual earnings for each individual in the scheme. Pension contributions to DC schemes vary, but are commonly between 10 per cent and 15 per cent, of which the employee will often pay only 5 per cent. His or her annuity is purchased on retirement at the time the pension is required. A large well known retail organisation recently changed from a DB to a DC scheme for all new entrants into which the employer now pays 5 per cent and the employee a minimum of 5 per cent. At the minimum, it is very unlikely that such a DC scheme would offer as good a pension as the predecessor DB scheme.

The SERPS scheme serves individuals who do not come within either the DB or DC categories. From time to time SERPS has changed in structure and is now complicated. Basically, the contributions to the scheme are linked to the earnings of an employee between a defined lower earnings limit and a defined upper earnings limit of National Insurance contributions. The pension earned is then 1.25 per cent of average earnings between these two limits for each year under the scheme; the best twenty years count for pension, i.e. a maximum of 25 per cent between the upper and lower earnings limits.

The government may well make other changes in SERPS and there have been suggestions from both major political parties that SERPS should be wound up. It is a pay-as-you-go unfunded scheme, which is difficult to drop without incurring major expense. Both major political parties would prefer some scheme that combined elements of both DB and DC schemes, but they are wary as to the costs and legal implications, as well as the lengthy period of change-over that would be involved.

The Pensions Act of 1995, which came into force in April 1997, codified earlier Acts and tightened up various regulations, especially those of DB schemes. In particular, the Act conferred further rights on employees with regard to past service. Membership is now voluntary for DB members, but they must join or retain one of the three options available. Past service in DB has, nowadays, to be maintained by the company as a deferred pension if the individual so wishes.

The May 1997 budget abolished the current tax rebates on investments in DB and DC schemes. For DB schemes this change is estimated to reduce the current annual investment rate from about 4.5 per cent to 4.0 per cent, a reduction of about 11 per cent. This cut the income of all funded DB pension schemes collectively by approximately £3.5 billion per annum. Such schemes are therefore likely to consider paring future benefits and/or encourage the movement from DB to DC schemes. An employer wishing to cut costs could close a DB scheme and set up a new DC scheme, or keep the DB scheme for existing members, starting a new DC scheme for new employees. If any such changes are made, individuals should ensure that all existing assets relating to DB benefits are ring-fenced.

Defined contribution scheme members have likewise been affected by the May 1997 budget. Employers pay into an individual's fund, to which the individual adds his or her own contributions. The promise does not relate directly to the size of pension, but to the size of the fund when he or she reaches retirement. This fund then pays an annuity for life. Employers have no obligation to top up any individual's fund if, for instance, investments do not perform as well as expected. The major Act change in the 1997 budget reduced the investment returns on money purchase schemes. Projected annuities (pensions) will fall unless individuals top them up with further contributions. Commentators have suggested that annuities will, in due course, fall by about 10–15 per cent unless extra contributions of about 1–2 per cent per annum of pay are made into the fund.

Another consequence of the 1997 abolition of dividend rebates for pension schemes is that many individuals may switch out of DB or DC schemes and move into SERPS. It will now be advantageous for all women and many men to stay in, or even return to, SERPS. Estimates of the cost to the government if the change is implemented range up to around £500 million per annum. The situation could be rectified if the rebate used to determine which individuals can be freed from SERPS grows by about a tenth to prevent major movements back into SERPS.

DIVORCE

For many years, irrespective of the various forms of pensioning, there has been considerable agitation as to the fairness of the procedures used to deal with pension rights when a divorce occurs. These rights may well be substantial but are, commonly, in the sole name of the husband. Moreover, if the pension rights are a major part of the accrued assets of a married couple, it has often been difficult to be seen to be fair to the two parties involved in a divorce.

In February 1997 the Conservative government published a White Paper suggesting how pensions might be split in order to have a more equitable arrangement between the two individuals concerned. The principle proposed involves pension rights being taken fully into account in the context of the overall financial situation of the divorcing couple, with a 'clean break' preferable whenever it can be appropriately made. The total value of the divorcing couple's existing pension rights should, as far as possible, be maintained when the split of overall assets is made.

The White Paper further proposed that divorced couples should not be placed in a more advantageous position than married couples, whilst other members of any pension scheme or schemes involved should not have to bear any extra financial expenses because of the split. The taxpayer should likewise be protected. Types of schemes to be considered in divorce proceedings could include:

- Occupational schemes (DB), including funded and unfunded approved schemes, and small self-administered schemes.
- Personal pension arrangements, money purchase schemes and retirement annuity contracts, including those of the self-employed (DC).
- Legislation that would enable the splitting of SERPS, where applicable, as part of the settlement.

The basic state retirement pension would not need to provide such splitting. This pension or pensions would be taken into account, together with other assets, with the income and benefits available to the divorcing couple when considering their overall financial position.

The government proposed that, when it is necessary to place a capital value on the pension rights of a scheme member, the method of valuing accrued private pension rights should be by the use of the cash equivalent transfer value (CETV). This is a well established and understood actuarial method, commonly used when scheme members transfer their DB pension rights from one scheme to another scheme. The method is, however, not accepted by everyone as completely fair, the unease being that the method tends to undervalue the assets held in the scheme of which the divorcee is a member. The value of the assets of the non-employee involved after the split may thereby be lower than expected. Clearly the implementation of such schemes is going to be complex in many situations. However, where there are substantial 'free' assets, the split may be relatively straightforward.

It is expected that most ex-wives will be better off than they would have been after divorce in earlier years, whilst the division of income between divorced partners should be more even than hitherto. The future income tax demands upon the combined divorcees will be lowered, estimated by the government to be of the order of £50 million per annum when the system has been running for some twenty years or so.

PENSION VALUE

The general view of pensioning has, over the years, aimed for a pension of some half the income level achieved at final salary. Current pension average level is already somewhat lower than the ideal average level. The value of the state retirement basic pension is steadily falling; SERPS likewise is falling in value over time in real terms. Hence it seems essential for the private sector to provide and manage most future pensioning arrangements. The mis-selling scandal has, unfortunately, led to personal pensions being treated very much as a second-class option. The consequence is that a new form of personal pension – along the government's stakeholder pension procedures – will perforce have to emerge. Moreover, stakeholding pensions will have to be at an appropriate level and additionally be made compulsory, whether the member is an employee or self-employed, if the appropriate required level of pensioning is to be achieved. Voluntary arrangements would leave a hostage to fortune for the next century.

LONG-TERM CARE

People live longer than hitherto, and so there is a greater need for long-term care in the community. Table 11.3 shows the Government Actuary's projection of the demographic breakdown of the future size and structure of the Great Britain population. The number of those of pensionable age is expected to rise from 10.3 million in 1990 to 15.3 million in 2050, a rise of nearly 50 per cent in the sixty-year period. More important, the ratio of those working to pensioners is expected to fall from 3.3 to 2.1 in the same period, demonstrating the pressure to shift the balance from those of 'working age' to those of 'retired age'. This demographic problem is not unique to the UK. Indeed, it is worse in many other countries, particularly some of those in the EU. France is a major case, with its allied pension arrangements heavily geared to the pay-as-you-go system.

At the same time it is clear that pensioners themselves are on average getting older, inevitably raising the number who need long-term care (LTC). Some 40 per cent of UK hospital and community health service expenditure in the NHS is currently spent on those aged sixty-five and above, a percentage that is expected to rise.

Table 11.3 Summary of 1991-based projection of GB population (million; percentage of totals in brackets)

Age group	1990	2000	2010	2030	2050
1 Children (0–15)	11.3	12.1	11.6	11.1	10.2
	(20.2)	(20.9)	(19.6)	(18.3)	(17.7)
2 Working ages					
(16–64 men,	34.4	35.2	36.0	33.7	32.1
16–59 women)	(61.4)	(60.9)	(60.8)	(55.9)	(55.8)
3 Pensionable ages	10.3	10.5	11.6	15.5	15.3
	(18.5)	(18.2)	(19.7)	(25.7)	(26.5)
Total	56.1	57.8	59.3	60.3	57.6
4 (2/3) Working ages/					
pensioners	3.3	3.3	3.1	2.2	2.1

Long-term care formally comes into operation where a person is unable to look after himself or herself, and needs care from others. Many taxpayers believe that they are automatically entitled to LTC, on the grounds that they have contributed through the tax and National Insurance systems during their working lives. Long-term care, however, has been means-tested ever since the 1948 National Assistance Act. If the public perception is different, that may be because LTC is commonly tied up with health care, which is basically free at the point of need. Inevitably, disappointed expectations regarding LTC have become a major political problem.

During the 1970s the funding of LTC for those who did not have enough income to pay for it themselves came from voluntary organisations, backed up by local authorities pressuring Social Security offices to make payments to individuals requiring LTC. There was informal means testing of any such payments.

In 1983 the system was further formalised, with social security payments to those who qualified on grounds of lack of income limited to those with total capital of less than £8,000. Full payment was made to those who had capital of less than £3,000. Care plans in local authority homes were financed, on a means-tested basis, by the appropriate local authority. Long-term care in NHS hospital beds, however, remained free. Thus, although LTC had always been provided on a means-tested basis, except in NHS beds, means testing became explicit under the changed financing arrangements.

The 1983 arrangements empowered those in need of LTC who were in receipt of social security to use a private, rather than a local authority, home. However, this change provided an incentive for the local authority to avoid the full range of domestic care services, which could be an efficient alternative to putting people into residential homes. The local authority generally did not recoup, through user charges, the full cost of domestic services. The new system improved the potential quality of the care environment for those individuals paid for by the state, creating further potential to erode the informal LTC sector and increasing public costs. It may also, via the Community Care Act 1990, have reduced the incentive to make more private provision, increasing the incentive to avoid the means test.

The 1990 Act, implemented in 1993, transferred to local authorities the portion of the social security budget which paid for the care element of LTC. It then became a cash limited grant, which could be spent on the provision of care at their own discretion. Under the Act, the local authority budget is to be spent on individuals according to their needs; costs can be recouped by local authorities from individuals, according to their means. The grant can be used to finance either domestic services or long-term residential care. The latter care can be in either local authority or private homes, the local authority being the contracting party.

The reality for those who do not 'pass' the social security means test is that they are likely to be asked to finance their care for themselves and receive no social security payments. This can happen even when the individual has a limited income should his total assets (including the primary residence if entering residential care) be above £16,000. Some contribution for the user is, however, required if assets are above £10,000.

Simply put, the alternatives in LTC policy are that either the state pays automatically for LTC or everyone is expected to save or insure for LTC. It is estimated that about one person in six who reaches the age of sixty will need LTC at some point later in his or her life. If it is to be left to the state the individual could – as is currently the case – suffer. If individuals decide to gamble on the possible need for LTC by making no provision, they are effectively gambling that, in the dire event of LTC becoming necessary, doctors and hospitals would not refuse to treat the elderly poor. The problem surrounding such a moral hazard could then raise its ugly head.

Many elderly individuals own a home and its value can, at least in theory, frequently yield sufficient cash from its sale to provide adequate LTC. Indeed, under current government policy, the state can recover costs of LTC through the sale of a house, with an obligation to cover the costs themselves only if the total available assets are less than £10,000. In many instances, however, the children may have expected to receive a legacy from their parents. Possible current scenarios for the problems arising that have been considered are:

- Reliance on the state. Currently the situation lies in the hands of local authorities who, usually, will give financial assistance only if total assets are below £10,000 (sometimes a limit of £16,000 is agreed).
- Costs taken out of personal income and savings. This is a possible option for some. Potential costs of an individual needing care can be up to approximately £17,000 annually. With inexorable inflation this could mean that even selling a house may not, in all instances, guarantee lifelong care. At some point the state may have to step in.

- Partner or relative looks after the needy person. This option is fraught with difficulties, e.g. the partner becomes increasingly frail, the elderly succumb to chronic illness such as Alzheimer's disease, etc.

None of these options is likely to provide the reassurance that most people want in extreme old age. A person's ability to remain independent would be jeopardised, assets and income threatened and, perhaps most important of all, relations with a partner or family could be seriously undermined.

Current arrangements for LTC do not involve public finance to anything like the same extent as the provision of health; but the balance of costs (whoever shoulders the burden of LTC) is going to grow. The means testing of public provision for LTC involves serious disincentives to saving. If people are to be encouraged to save for their old age to pay for their care, whilst at the same time those who do not save still get the same care at public expense, the implied return on savings could be minus 100 per cent! Four approaches have been put forward to satisfy future LTC requirements:

- Individuals should themselves build up over time enough resources, via pension income, investment savings and property, to pay for care directly or, alternatively, be able to purchase an annuity to cover the liabilities.
- Insurance mechanisms could be used to cover the required costs of LTC. An LTC insurance plan would enable a person to choose how and where he or she will be cared for, retaining some income and assets intact. Most important, it would enable a person to preserve his or her independence and respect the family's inheritance. The National Association of Pension Funds in 1996 gave some appropriate cost estimates. An appropriate *single* premium paid at the age of sixty would be approximately £15,000 for a man and £24,000 for a woman. The premium would be higher if the individual took out the policy at a later age. If the individual wished to pay *annual* premiums from age sixty the cost would be approximately £1,300 per annum for a man, £1,900 for a woman. The single and annual premiums would then both be smaller than the quoted figures, if the policies were to be taken out at an earlier age.
- A third option involves a form of lien on a house owned by an individual (or a married couple), written in such a way that the elderly individual, or married couple, agrees with an appropriate

insurer to allow a claim on some proportion of the value of their dwelling in return for providing cover for LTC. Such an insurance policy avoids the present inheritance lottery, which lies behind the strong feelings generated when housing wealth is used to finance LTC.

- A further option derives from a Joseph Rowntree Foundation report which advocated the introduction of a compulsory National Care Insurance Scheme along the lines of the German system of compulsory insurance. The Rowntree report espoused the idea that employees and the self-employed should be required to make an annual National Care Insurance contribution of 1.5 per cent of their earnings within the lower and upper National Insurance earnings limits. This option is approximately equivalent to an average 0.8 per cent of gross earnings, a figure that is somewhat higher than the contribution rate suggested by the National Association of Pension Funds under the second proposal above.

Most people wish to enjoy independence and take for granted the right to decide how and when they should spend their earnings and savings. For those who need care in later life, lack of independence comes at a point in their life when they are at their most vulnerable. Losing one's independence is a sobering experience. Relying upon favours and living by the rules of others hold little attraction.

Will LTC remain a complex set of arrangements in which there is a mixture of private and public money involving complex means-tested procedures, or will individuals be left to make their own provision? Or, finally, will they have to rely on a compulsory tax for those in work to pay in advance for all LTC? The government has proposed a Royal Commission on LTC. The terms of reference are 'to work out a fair system for the funding of long-term care for the elderly' – a proposal from the Labour manifesto of 1 May 1997. Governmental changes in pension arrangements could well be entwined with LTC, and an integrated and acceptable view of all forms of social insurance must surely be the aim for the twenty-first century. The present chapter has shown how ambitious that is.

REFERENCE

Bos E., Vu M. T., Massiah E. and Bulatao R. A. (1994) *World Population Projects 1994–95*, World Bank, Washington, D.C.

INDEX